I0423040

Sophie L. Barnes : contact@helpheretoday.com
www.helpheretoday.com

First Printing: January 2013
Second Printing: March 2014

ISBN- ISBN-13: 978-1482032093
ISBN-10: 1482032090

This book is dedicated to my biggest fan and supporter, my husband, Peter.

Praises about this book

By Ez

With plenty of years of experience, Sophie knows how to break down the do's and don'ts of weight management and thoroughly explains why we tend to spiral into the same routines over and over.

She makes it so clear and easy to follow and uses personal life experience to demonstrate her theories. I love that this book tackles body image, not from a physical point of view, but from a mental and emotional state of mind! Sophie challenges us to dig deep and find the root cause of our habits and helps realize and turn them into positive changes that LAST!

Personally, I found this book to help me also deal with other emotional issues in my life that have been lingering on for a while.

A must read!

By Cathy -
Sophie takes you down her own personal weight loss journey and leads by example. Her struggles are inspirational and motivate you to take the small but necessary steps to improve your own life; body, mind and spirit. What I really loved was that she included key questions in each chapter to get you thinking about your own weight loss issues and the obstacles that have prevented you from your reaching your goals in the past.

I highly recommend this book and her website HelpHereToday.com for anyone who has seen those hard lost pounds slowly creep back on as a perfect companion to help find lasting success.

By **Judes**

Courage and perseverance are the two words that pop into my head after reading this book. It takes courage to talk about one's own personal ups and downs in a book for everyone else to read. It also takes perseverance to always want to continue after falling down or realizing that what we are doing is just not working for us, and that something has to change.

The only person who can make those changes is yourself. It inspires us to tackle our own demons and face them head on. Deep down, we all know that these demons will always be there until we decide to do something about them. Facing our fears to confront the unknown is always scary but once we have gone over the first hurdle, it is that first stepping stone that gives us the courage to continue tackling all of the other fears that we have.

Sophie shows us that anyone can do that by staying true to ourselves.

By **Nathalie**

Sophie's book is really fun to read, having put real stories makes it an easy read. The topics are really about things that affect us personally and I was totally addicted to reading it non-stop. I myself used the chapter for not gaining weight on vacation and it worked, I did not gain a pound. I was very happy because I always take an average of 5 pounds per week of vacation. So I say thank you Sophie!

I was not convinced that taking the time and write in my journal was useful, but I realized that stopping and taking a step back from our daily lives is really good and our sub-

conscious is more likely to reveal our deepest secrets and revelations when we do it regularly. I have started that step.

I set goals such as suggested in Sophie's book and it works perfectly ... I feel really motivated to do them and it seems that it allowed me to have a better focus on my goals and I'm better equipped to move in direction I want.

Again, thank you for these guidelines; they really helped me develop myself further. I am now very happy. I feel better about myself. For sure I still have work to do with my behavior with food, but I am on the right path and I feel great.

Content

Introduction

No one can make you feel inferior without your consent.

ELEANOR ROOSEVELT
First lady of the United States from 1933 to 1945
and wife of Franklin Delano Roosevelt

You have reached your goal weight. You were thrilled for about a second and a half. All that hard, consistent work, and now what? You did not get the dreamy boyfriend, the fantastic job, the modeling contract, or that shot at acting or singing you always wanted. You did not get discovered, you know, like you hear sometimes: "I was just walking down the street and I got discovered!"

So really, at this point you are thinking, "What was all this for?" Happiness? Peace of mind? To lose that loser feeling you had when you were fat? Did you hope to lose the anxiety of clothes shopping, dating, and doing job interviews? Did you think you'd reach a point where how much you weighed would not define how well you felt?

Oh God, I know! It all sounds so familiar! Do you realize that when I write in my journal, next to the date, I put my weight? Yes! Pathetic. Sad, really. For so long, my weight defined who I was. So I lost the weight, but then I had all those feelings you are having. My biggest fear was that I might gain it back. And, of course, when you focus on that, guess what happens? I had a big event in my life this past year, my wedding. Over eight months before the wedding, I embarked on a health regimen with a nutritionist and a private trainer. I lost 25 pounds in time for the wedding. Three months later, I had gained 10 pounds back. Fourteen months later, I was 10 pounds higher than when I embarked on my health regimen. I had thought that I had broken my yo-yo weight cycle. I had lost the weight in a healthy way, so why was it coming back?

Gaining the weight back was one thing, but my biggest annoyance was that I had not reached the peace of mind in my relationship with food that I thought I would have at a certain weight (or age!). I realized that whatever baggage (yes pun intended!), I carried around at my fattest, it was still with me at my thinnest. Unless I was able to put that baggage down, it was going to bring me right back there, to my fattest and most miserable.

I did not want that. I never wanted that. I was so tired of knowing how I was doing by how I was eating. So I decided to write this book. Why? Because I needed to find out, for real, what to do next. I just couldn't believe that after reaching my ideal weight before the wedding, my first impulse was to have a big meal as a celebration! It seemed that I did not believe for one second that I belonged at that weight. I am not giving you that weight number on purpose because that number is different for everyone. What is important is that I was at my goal weight. In retrospect, I felt like Oprah must have felt when she did that liquid diet and stayed at that weight for less than twenty-four hours, even if I had lost the weight in a healthy way.

I had my ups and downs in those eight months with the nutritionist and trainer. I always had to fight those inner (or outer) voices that told me that I could have that extra dessert. The problem with me is that I cannot have one dessert. I cannot have three potato chips; I need a big bag or at least two small bags. And I need two or three chocolate bars. I am an all-or-nothing kind of a girl. Those who binge know what I am talking about. As a side note, I don't purge (but I used to), and for those who do, you need to get professional help. It is damaging your body. In these moments, it felt like another part of me had taken over. That self was insecure, anxious, and hurt, and in order to avoid those feelings, we have to fill in the bucket with our escape mechanism, for me, through junk food. For others, it may be drugs or alcohol. A question that this raises is why it is so important to avoid those feelings. Do they really hurt that bad? Are they so painful? Today, my answer is "No!"

When I force myself to listen and feel, I find that these feelings aren't so bad. So why have I been avoiding them all my life? I believe that what I was afraid of was that those miserable feelings I was experiencing would last forever, so I ate. Well, I am not a therapist, but I have seen one for many years, so I assume that if you have these bad feelings you were probably young when you first experienced the pain, and it was earth shattering painful, and you relive that memory every time those emotions or feelings come around.

I have noticed that when I let those feelings go unchecked, meaning that I just eat tons of junk food to bury the feelings, I get numb. I disappear. Then I feel disgusted with myself. But, oh good news, when I don't allow myself to fall into the binging habit, I sit, I listen, and I feel. And it feels nice to have me listening to me for a change.

My husband calls me "ma petite gourmande." I enjoy food. I enjoy all the desserts and pasta dishes and croissants and Danishes and muffins and warm bread and butter. I love them. I probably should never move to France or Italy. Don't they have the best pastries and pasta dishes? But I have to be mature and choose the food that is best for my body and my overall health. I don't always do that. The internal fight has been going on forever, really. I cannot tell you exactly when it started. In my teens, I guess. I have just started to understand what the fight has been really about. And that's why I am writing this book. I think it can help others find solutions as well.

The idea of this book came to me one morning when I was writing in my journal and I was thinking, well I have lost the weight, but now what? I didn't feel any happier, and I had already started gaining some of the weight back and I wondered where I had gone wrong.

This book is not meant to be read and put on a shelf. It is meant to be your companion to help you succeed. You will want to take it out again and again for very specific needs. You will have some homework to do, where you will have to sit down and think and write and take action. Taking action is important. I have read many self-help books and listened to inspirational CDs, and watched *The Oprah Show* and the OWN network, but I didn't know how to apply all this information I had in my head. So this book is a collection of tricks, exercises, and experiences that I hope will help you as it has helped me.

While reading this book you will have to spend some time analyzing yourself. Who is running the show? Who are you? Are you a strong individual with a strong self-image? Are you sometimes strong, sometimes weak? Does your younger self come out at the least opportune times? Do you have internal fights about what you want and what is best for you? You need to answer these questions to find out who you are at a basic level. I firmly believe that unless you discover these answers for yourself, you will never conquer your relationship with food. The internal fight between the one who wants to be healthy and strong and the one who wants to remain the victim of your past will continue. Doesn't that sound exhausting? Don't you want to spend all that energy doing something rewarding for you and your life instead? So ask yourself why you want to lose weight. Really, why? That answer will guide your next steps.

One of the most important first steps forward involves changing your perception of yourself. Do you realize you are carrying around with you a perception that is 10 or 20 or 30 years old? Isn't it time to upgrade? The story of you needs a change. When you were young, people might have said that you were the fat, ugly kid, or the lazy kid, or the dumb kid. Whatever your story was, you can change it. Create a new story for yourself. In the chapters to come, there will be discussions and guidance on how to work with patterns and beliefs to help you accomplish your goals. These patterns and beliefs guide your every move and I bet you barely notice them!

Changing perception also means reviewing your thoughts. They are the first words anyone hears, and, as Maya Angelou said, they do eventually turn into action. What you think of yourself today will become who you are tomorrow, so it is important to have the right thoughts that will bring you to where you want to be.

There are some simple tools that you will need to have; you'll need to write in your journal consistently and imagine your future. Nothing is just going to fall into your lap. Prepare the future you want with clean and precise actions. Why wait until you have it to act like you have it? Let's act *as-if* now.

Look around you. Do you have some cleaning to do? Everyone does. In order to become who you want to be you have to do a big spring cleaning. That involves all area of your life: your job, your relationships, your environment, and, of course, your closets.

A lot of my energy used to be spent on guilt and worry. I wanted to use my energy more efficiently so I added a chapter about those feelings. A lot of time can be spent on guilt and worry, and they can be killers; they kill energy, hope, and the natural flow of your being. In order to achieve overall well-being, it is important to spend some time clearing out everything that prevents you from being your best self.

Meditation and visualization are also important tools to have. You don't have to move to India for six months to experience the benefits of it. In order to change, you need to believe. You need to believe in yourself first, and you need to believe that life or the Universe will answer. The Universe will change around you to meet your new you. I find that meditating and visualizing helps accomplish peace of mind, helps to focus on what I want, and helps me to believe.

I also have chapters on the all-important topics of forgiveness and faith. The two became very clear to me on my quest to clear some old wounds. Forgiveness is an amazing concept, and if done properly, it can free you. And it feels amazing. When I talk about faith, I am not talking about religion. I am talking about the kind of faith that makes you believe in yourself and believe you can achieve what you want, no matter what.

Considering that I went through a big life event and soon after started gaining weight, I thought it would be important to talk about not losing your focus after big life events. But keeping focus also means not letting day-to-day life and everyday problems distract you from your goals. These little problems and stresses can kill your dreams and goals. You have to find time every day to take some form of action towards them. This will help keep you focused.

And you thought you were just losing weight!

Chapter 1: Who is Running the Show?

There are seeds of self-destruction in all of us that
will bear only unhappiness if allowed to grow.

DOROTHEA BRANDE
A well-respected writer and editor

It is 14 months today that we got married. It has been amazing; we love calling each other husband and wife. Now we are back to reality and back to work, and I am back to worrying about my weight. I gained the 25 pounds back plus 10, and since I did not gain weight on the honeymoon, it is really after that, that it happened. Now I am back to square one.

I did not solve the problem that made me eat junk food. I am still anxious, nervous, frustrated, and dissatisfied with my life. I have been down lately. I have great moments of joy in my days, but also moments of feeling down. It is as if a part of me does not believe I deserve what I have, so I am trying to sabotage it. I was trying to figure out what occurred in my life in the past few months that activated a part of me that does not believe I deserve the best, and I think I figured out what it was. My father got sick, and he passed away not too long ago. I was in contact with people who knew me when I was young and insecure. Normally, I try to stay surrounded by people who belong in my present and not in my past, but sometimes, you know, the past catches up to you!

For six months, there was increased communications and visits with family. All the intensive face-to-face communications with some of the folks I had put behind me forced me to face some long hidden feelings. And I handled it by eating my way through it. This event totally reactivated a part of my self that I thought I had resolved—I guess life thought otherwise. It gave me a challenge and I failed! I am trying to be grateful when things like this happen because it forces me to face head on what I am trying to solve. And I know that if I don't solve it, it will keep coming back until I do.

So here I am getting down to the core of my problem, and my problem is not the chip or the chocolate bar; my problem is why do I need to eat so urgently when in distress? My reaction to stress is always the same. My adult self disappears to give all the space to my younger self. It annoys me that I let it happen. I let my world be run by an eight year old. Yes, I have determined that this part of my self that is hurt and frightened is eight years old. I have no scientific facts to base this on; it is a gut feeling. Also, the fact that starting my ninth year I had two major physical problems tends to tell me I am right that my eighth year was difficult.

When my younger self takes charge, my world becomes depressing and sad with no hope for escape. I have no doubt that this is how I felt when I was young. When my current self is in charge—the self who is more self-assured, more in control, feels more self-love, and who feels that I have choices—then my world is full of possibilities. I have found love with a great husband, good coworkers, and great friends. When I am centered in my core, I am master of my domain. I build my dream board, I plan my goals, I eat right, I exercise, and life is great. I am not trying to separate myself into multiple people, but I firmly believe that I have within me a small version of me who is stuck in time. She is still there in pain and afraid, and she feels stuck in her circumstances. Every once in a while, an event will occur to wake her up. I am fairly strong-minded and pig-headed so we inevitably end up wrestling.

To wake up my eight-year-old frame of mind, I have to activate a pattern, which is that I think very negatively. I build up the negative side of everything in my life. I build up the pain, the anger, the anxiety, and the feeling that I am a loser and will never accomplish anything worthy. I build all that up and then I act it as if my world were hopeless, with no way out, exactly like I thought it was back then. So instead of living in the present and being at my goal weight, happy and content, I suddenly act as if I were everything to the contrary. I knew about using "act-as-if" to improve your life, but I never in my dreams thought I was using it to bring my life down!

This makes so much sense. All these years, I was trying to figure out why I was disappearing so easily behind a part of my self that should not exist anymore. When I was saying I couldn't move on until I resolved this, I was right. As long as I play the role of the victim in my head, I cannot move on to be anything else. So all those goals and dreams will not happen until I let go and release this part of my self that insists on remaining stuck in time.

I never understood when people told me that I didn't have money or success because I didn't feel I deserved it. You see, I felt I did deserve it. One hundred percent of me at a given time believes in me. I did not understand when they said I didn't feel I deserved it because I did and I was doing all the right things. But then my young self kicks in. She is not "awake" or there 20-30% of the time at all times. That is not how it works. When she appears, she takes up 100% of the space. She wants the entire stage. And my adult self disappears.

I've also found that if one day my younger self takes over, then the next day it gets easier for her to do it and the next day even easier. And she stays for longer, too. Today is one hour, tomorrow will be two. The down feeling I have afterwards happens because when my adult self gets back in charge I am thinking, "What the heck just happened?" It is exactly the same as if I were looking at a child who did something stupid: I can't believe that kid just did that! Now, as an adult, I have to rebuild my hopes, trust, and faith. The thing is, my younger self now has momentum and strength; she had her moment of fame and space, and she wants more. That is when the internal fight begins between the two of us.

When I am not completely in charge, I feel my young hurt self, and I can see that when I focus on my goals and I associate negative feelings to them. For example, I imagine myself rich and living in a luxurious condo in San Diego. Then very quickly, I have the image of a relative showing up wanting money and fighting with me. I bring on a negative feeling and associate it to being rich. That is why I was not rich! Remember when I said I did not understand when people told me that I was not 100% committed to being rich? Well, here is the explanation.

My adult side could not understand the logic because she felt that I was 100% committed. However, the thing is, so is my younger self. She is a ball of pure, raw emotion. Anything she does is associated with emotion and makes her ten times stronger. I can repeat my affirmation to be rich 20 times a day, but as soon as negative emotions are linked to it via my younger self then it all goes down the drain. I unwillingly associated bad things to being rich. It would be easier not to be rich. Then, I wouldn't have to worry about fights over money. Very eight-year-old thinking, don't you agree? This is why I say, as long as you carry around these distorted emotions, you will never move on.

Now, I mentioned being rich, but what about being fat? Could it be that I associate more pain with being thin then with being fat? Is that why I regained the weight? I picked my brains again and again to get at that truth. I kept telling myself there was no way I felt being thin was painful. But yes, I did. It is binary; it is a yes and no thing. I associated being thin and beautiful to being an easy target for abusive guys. I needed the junk food because it rid myself of that bad feeling in that specific moment: it was more painful to remain thin and not have the junk food then to have it.

Well, now that we know that, what do we do? Think about the times when your adult self succeeded in not letting your younger self take over. How did you do that? Find out and do it again and again. I find that as you grow older and slowly get stronger (through therapy or self-help books or self-analysis), you begin to enjoy who you are. You feel stronger, happier, believe more in yourself, and have hopes and dreams that become more and more daring. You come to have bigger and bigger goals. When you grow stronger, you have no patience for your younger side who is sad, anxious, and angry. You become intolerant with your self.

That is where I am; I have no patience for my younger self anymore. She no longer belongs to who I am today. I want to let her go. And if you are reading this, I think you are ready to let your younger self go, too. Now, how do you do that?

WITH LOVE

With love and tenderness. First of all, it is a part of me that suffered. I was scared, hurt and had huge anxiety. I had a hard time falling asleep all my life, until I met my husband. The anxiety level in me has always been huge, and now I am starting to understand why. My younger self was trying to speak out, to let me know that a part of myself was still there and still existed.

So step one is to acknowledge her. It is important to acknowledge that she is part of me and still exists, and that she still hurts and my adult self needs to take care of her and love her.

Then I needed to find out what wakes her up. Why is she manifesting herself one day and not the next? The answer I found was feelings! Simple feelings. In my case, it may be a feeling of hurt, a feeling of being stuck in a bad situation, a feeling of desperation or hopelessness or being unloved, feeling like a loser, or even feeling general anxiety. Any feelings that I felt when I was in that place that is stuck in time will bring me back to that time. And the amazing thing with feelings? No matter how many years have passed since then, they communicate with each other (past and present) faster than the speed of light.

Having to be in close contact again with all members of my family brought back my younger self in full force. I could not control her anymore. For weeks, she took over, and I ate junk food and pushed away exercise. Every day I would wake up with the hope that I was back in charge. But I wasn't. I was not able to take charge of myself. So how did I finally do it?

The next step is to cut the cord that tied me to that time because it was not my reality anymore. I am not saying I will never feel hurt or hopelessness again. What I am saying is when I do, it does not have to send me into a tailspin of the awfulness I felt back then. I wanted to retrieve those feelings into my present, and experience it now with my current reality.

I sat and talked to my younger self who was trying to take over and explained that the past did not exist anymore. Have moments of love and understanding for what she was trying to grasp. She was only trying to do what she knows. Slowly and surely with soft discipline, I explained that it was time for her to let go of that pain. The poor, hurt sweetie needed to rest. Can you imagine the years of pain she has suffered through that clouded reality, reliving those awful feelings over and over again every year since they initially happened? Wasn't it time to let go? I wanted to let go of the pain, the anxiety, the hurt, the anger, the sadness, the feeling of pure fear grabbing at your throat and your stomach like there was no way out. Yes, I said it was time. I let it go. I am not saying I let her go; I am saying I let go of her pain.

Another lesson I learned was to change my physiology, as Tony Robbins[1] says. He notes that when you are about to get depressed, down, or feel victimized, your body takes on a certain position: hunched over, head down, frowning, hands by your side and not smiling. The fastest way to change that is to stand up, shake yourself, put your shoulders back, stand tall, and put a big smile on your face as if you could take on the world. This will affect your mental focus. Because they are aligned, if you change your physiology, you mind has no other option but to follow.

WHY?

Now, before you do anything, you need to understand why you keep this part of yourself around. You know it is not helping you grow to be a better person, you know it drags you down, so why carry it with you all these years? The answer is fear and habit. You are afraid to let go of that pain. It is familiar, and releasing it will make you lose an important part of yourself. You have been living with that side of yourself for so many years, how do you live without it? That is the fear of the unknown and the fear of change talking. So how do you address those fears? How do you change? That is what this book is about, and all the tricks and tools are coming up.

First, I believe you need to understand where your pain comes from, and second, you need to decide that staying in that victimized mode is more painful for you then changing. It took years to get to where you are. You now feel you have reached a point where you are strong enough to do it, so let's

---

[1] Tony Robbins, *Personnel Power*.

do it. One step at a time. Don't forget that your goal is to let go of the pain that you have associated with a part of you that is stuck in time; that part that makes you live today's events through the hurt of the past.

In order to release this part of you properly, you have to do it with love, forgiveness, and tenderness, but also strength: leave no option but to let go. That part of you will fight to stay. You have to be 100% committed to succeed in letting go of the pain. Your goal of being at peace with food, to no longer binge out your emotions, and to succeed at looking great and feeling great will not happen, will never happen, unless you release the part of you that is hurt. This is why you have to be 100% committed. Life knows you are getting geared up for this challenge, and it will give you plenty of opportunities to test your resolve. It will throw at you everything it can to see if you are ready to succeed.

Every morning, one of my affirmations is:

I am grateful for today and its challenges
that I overcome in order to get closer to my goal.

NOW WHAT?

So now that you understand where you are, let's see how to resolve it. Let's take an example. You get up in the morning, you work out, meditate, write in your journal, and you are ready to take on the world. You get to the office, your boss yells at you for a major mistake you made that cost the company tons of money. Ok, this is the first test of the day. How will you handle it? Will your stay centered with your adult as master of your domain and evaluate the situation calmly? Or will you let your younger self take over and react to today's events like a neurotic, self-destroying, sabotaging, throwing-a-tantrum kid? Well, when you put it like that!

The key to success is to NEVER let your younger self take over 100%. I know, easier said than done. Stop and listen. Go inward. If you feel your younger self flaring up, start to speak to your younger self right away. How does it feel? Personally, I get stomach pangs. I start feeling anxious, (actually uncontrolled anxiety) and if it is early morning, I desperately want a Danish and a coffee or if it is afternoon, chips and chocolate. And of course, I start my pattern of negative thinking and my physiology changes. If you find yourself in this position, what do you do?

The first thing to figure out is your pattern. Now that I know what mine is, I need to do two things. First I need to resolve the source of the problem, which is: wrongly handling today's situation with my young self instead of my grown self. I need to calm my younger self down. In Chapter 2, we will look at how to change a pattern, but for now, what you need to know is how to address that hurt, younger self that wants to take over.

You need to imagine talking to a child and approach your younger self with understanding and assurance: "I understand that you are hurt. That was pretty awful what was just said. Let me dig into this problem, logically. I will analyze it and see what happens." Your younger self needs to feel security. When your younger self flares up like that, it is because there is a feeling of being attacked. No way. Your adult self is there to protect all of you no matter what. The sooner all your selves get that, the better you (and everyone!) will feel. At times, your younger self will try to overtake you. This is when soft (and sometimes hard) discipline comes in. You have to stand your ground and make it clear that you are not going anywhere. Your younger self needs to take a back seat and let you do your job. Think about the double fights that you have had to deal with all your life. As an adult, you have to contain the current situation, but at the same time, you have this side of you who just wants to have a tantrum and walk away because she is hurt (in this case walk away from the job!). You have always had to deal with two things at the same time, but that is not how adults deal with rough situations and your younger self needs to understand this. The stronger your adult and your core become, the less space your hurt younger self will take up.

Take action:

> But at the same time, keep in mind that your young self is hurt. She is re-living a past event. You need to consciously relive it with her. So while you are taking charge at work, take some time on a quiet morning and write in your diary and try to figure out where this pain comes from. You need to simulate that event or similar events to bring this pain to the surface and relive it properly; that means reliving the pain with who you are today. It may be painful but it will relieve so much old bundled up pain that after you have done it, you will feel relieved and re-energized.

> The next time someone attacks you, this old pain will not resurface because you took care of it.

I find that I am in control most of the time, but I also find that now, when my younger self comes out, she is more angry and anxious than she used to be. This makes it harder for me to control her, but it is also a good thing. It means that I am headed in the right direction. When you get to this point, you'll find that the challenges are tougher, but as you conquer them, you get closer and closer to being free. Keep doing the exercise of writing down your pain and simulating it as if it was happening for real. Do it for each pain and relieve each and everyone of them, one at the time.

Stay strong, stay on top, and don't forget to get physical. I like to go for walks or climb stairs in my building in order to reconnect with my body and feel strong. I come back, my head high, shoulders back, and I'm smiling. Keep 100% committed; nothing else matters. Until this is solved, nothing you want will happen.

If the anxiety is still there, that means you have not yet resolved the pain she is suffering from. Go back to simulating events. You know you are on the right path when you feel it in your gut. To prevent your younger self from taking all the space, she needs to realize that you are now ready to be there and help her let go of the pain. The hurt can be released, and your younger self can now rest or come out and play instead. All she really wants is to be listened to!

You cannot change the circumstances of the past. You can only change your reactions to it with your reality of today. This is what people mean when they say; "it is your choice". What happened then was not your choice, your reactions then as a child were the best you could do at that time. But what you do today as an adult is your choice. Do you want to remain angry, sad, and anxious forever? Do you want that to define you? Do you want to keep on being the victim? Is that how you want to be remembered?

You, today, define who you are and who you chose to be. It is your choice. Rewrite your own story on how You want it to be. If you are reading this book, it is because a large part of you is ready to let go. That is great news. So buckle up, it will be quite a ride. One event at a time, one hour at a time, one day, one week, one month at a time. Be persistent and never give up. You, all of you, are worth it. The more you stay centered and strong, the more you will be releasing that part of yourself that is hurt and needs to rest. But be careful. Just when you think you have it all figured out and have it all together: Bang! Another test will come your way. Maybe a bigger one. Stay focused, and stay in a place of love and forgiveness and strength instead of anger and anxiety. You need to gain momentum. Take action. The minute you sit back and do nothing, that is when your younger self will take over.

The death of my father forced me to face some events of the past. My mother died three years ago, and, back then, I was not ready to face anything. I re-entered the family with huge cement walls all around me. No windows or doors for communication. And, of course, someone said something that hurt me to the core and that reminded me why I didn't want to be there in the first place. When I returned to my family again this year, I was more open and strong. I actually approached that sibling who had said something hurtful, and he did not remember it. I had let it sit like a stain on my heart for three years and he did not even remember it. Unbelievable! After I analyzed the situation, it became clear. People have their own issues to deal with, and often they attack because they are hurting themselves; it really has nothing to do with you.

Seeing this and reviewing some events, I realized that my perception of some of those events was tainted by my own hurt, fear and anxiety. I am not saying I dreamt the whole thing. It was and felt very real. How many times have I hurt my younger brother with my words and actions even though I love him dearly! At this point, I realized that I did not want to continue my life with this anger.

The last time I saw my father, towards the end, I told him "I forgive you" and "I love you". And I meant it. In the past few months that he was in the hospital, he shared some of his fears, goals and dreams that he hadn't accomplished in his lifetime. That information shone a new light on why he had sometimes behaved in ways that were extremely hurtful to me.

As I am about to conclude this chapter, I ask myself, why I want to lose weight. My answer is that I do not want to lose weight. What I want is to treat myself with love and respect. I want to be happier in my own skin. I want to grow and follow my dreams. I want to hang on to my hopes and believe that they are possible. You know those days where you feel completely centered and strong? I want more and more of those days. I want to surround myself with people who believe in me, love me, and push me to be more and better. I want to get up in the morning excited at life. That is what I want. What do you want? Why do you want to lose weight?

Chapter 1 Summaries

- ➤ Why do you want to lose weight?
- ➤ What activates your desire to eat junk food?
- ➤ What are the feelings you are trying to cover up with junk food?
- ➤ Go back in time. What started this behavior?
- ➤ Review the steps to start managing your hurt self.

Chapter 2: Change Your Perception of Yourself

Insanity: doing the same thing over and over
again and expecting different results.

ALBERT EINSTEIN
German-born theoretical physicist who
developed the theory of general relativity

WHAT'S NEXT?

Calming down your hurt self is one thing. Now we need to ensure that your mechanisms to deal with today's life are healthy and strong. You built your mechanisms when you were young, and there is no reason why you can't change them and build better ones for today's reality. Some years from now, you might have to adjust them again. Sometimes, I find the perception I have of myself is negative: I am ugly, I am a loser, I am poor, I am not intelligent. This perception is buried deep inside me and every once in a while it comes out and affects my life negatively. I have been able to fight it off a lot. I have accomplished great things in my life. But I am tired of fighting with myself. I want to unite all my selves and move in one direction. I want my core self to be strong, self-assured, and energized. To do this, I need to change the perception I have of myself.

So yes, your adult, grounded self needs to take charge, but how? The problem I had when I lost the weight was that I did not change. Not really. Not in my core. My outside appearance changed but not who I really was. And who I believed I was got me fat in the first place. I needed to realize that first and foremost. You can try to ignore those voices deep inside you; you can say affirmations all day long, but they won't work. If you are here, it is because you managed to lose the weight without changing why you gained it in the first place. That in itself is amazing!

My wedding was coming up. As any women will tell you, that is a major event. I wanted to look my best. Most of the time during that period the adult self won. I had a goal. I had a dress I needed to fit into. My vanity dictated that I wanted to look my best at my wedding. That was the reality, and that was why I succeeded at losing the weight. So I lost the weight, but I did not focus on the reasons why I had gained the weight in the first place or why I wanted to eat bad food. Each person is different, and the reasons why people eat food they know is bad for them may differ, but one thing is true in all situations—it is less painful to eat junk food than to deal with what is happening.[2] The pain of thinking that I'd be at the altar with my soon to be husband in a plus-sized wedding dress was greater than the day-to-day pain I was experiencing that would normally have sent me to seek solace in junk food. I am an emotional eater. I eat when I am alone and sad, I eat when I am anxious or bored, and I eat when I am celebrating.

WHO IS RESPONSIBLE?

The first thing to do is take 100% responsibility for your life. You might want to read the first chapter of an amazing book I have read a few times.[3] The Success Principle from Jack Canfield. Since we are focusing on your relationship with food, then that is what we'll talk about but you can imagine that it is applicable to all areas of your life. I was at my goal weight about two months before the wedding. Then I was asked to take charge of major short-term project at work that had high visibility with upper-management. It was extremely stressful.

---

[2] Antony Robbins: Personal Power.
[3] Jack Canfield "The success principle."

I could have handled it with calmness and grace, but, no, I chose the rougher road. I had to work seven days a week, often from 7 a.m. to 11 p.m. with a few nights up in between. I blamed all kinds of people for my stress and my inability to handle it properly. I gave myself all kinds of permissions to eat all the wrong food and not work out because of it. I gained about ten pounds once again. I was understandably upset, but I did make those choices. Was it really someone else's fault that I ate so much chocolate and so many french fries? No, it was my choice. What you do today is your choice. Not some of the time but all of the time. You can blame your past, blame the people who hurt you in your past and who made you develop those bad habits or patterns that saved you then but are harming you now. But why allow those people or events run your life so many years later? I don't know about you, but I got tired of it. Why should I allow them to live rent-free in my head? I decided to stop them. That was a turning point for me. And if you are not willing to take charge of your life and stop blaming others, then close this book and go get a box of donuts. This is a showstopper to your success. Without taking charge of your life, you'll never find success.

PATTERNS

As I have mentioned, I have a pattern. In order for me to lose my adult control, I have to let my younger self put negative thoughts into my head: "victim," "guilt," "not loved," or "not good enough." That is how it starts for me. I build a whole scenario in my head. And I have a great imagination, so my sad scenario can go on forever and the feelings attached to it just grow and grow. As soon as I see this pattern starting, however, what I need to do is to stop it. Immediately! Antony Robbins', *Personal Power* talks about how to change patterns, and I encourage you to check them out.

Is there a pattern in your life that was not good for you that you changed? There was for me. When I was very young, I used to suck my thumb. My mother tried all kinds of ways to get me to stop sucking my thumb. You know what did it? Classmates started making fun of me at school. Sucking my thumb displeased my parents, but it gave me comfort and pleasure. Knowing it displeased my parents was not a strong enough feeling to stop me. But when my classmates started making fun of me, I felt pain. Enough pain to counteract the good feeling I was getting from doing it. What do you think happened? I stopped. I was not getting a good feeling from it anymore. I had associated pain with sucking my thumb, and I stopped. Once I associated pain to this bad pattern, it was easy to stop. Back then, I had not read or heard about how to stop patterns; it was just natural. So today, with all the knowledge that I now have, shouldn't it be easier? I guess it depends on how ready I am to get rid of a pattern. Some patterns may be harder to get rid of then others, but what I know for sure is that I need to link pain to it to get rid of it. If I am hanging on to a bad pattern, it is because I link pain to changing it; I am not ready to change it.

Let's look at the following example:

Your boss reprimands you on some work you potentially did not do to the best of your abilities. Either he tells you outright or uses passive aggressive methods to let you know he's unhappy with you.

Boy! With my desire to please, that would send me into a tailspin! Here is what would happen with my old process: First, my anxiety level would increase. I would repeat his negative statement or attitude over and over in my head. My first desire would be to get some junk food because, knowingly or not, I would now feel like a loser. My body would suddenly hunch over. Then I would get defensive. I would start attacking in my head everything and everyone that I felt was responsible for everything that did not work in my life. However, even if this seems like I was on the attack, I would still feel like a loser because I would not be looking at the core of the problem. All this would occur in a matter of minutes.

When something big happens, it is even more important to take time alone to analyze the situation as soon as you can, to logically try to keep the affects from taking over. What is dangerous for me is when I don't pay attention. I think I am a grown woman, and I try not to let it affect me. But then it grows on me like a shadow; it takes over and—boom—my adult self disappears and my younger self is suddenly taking up all the space inside me.

Still thinking of this work scenario, here are some questions to ask yourself based on whether you did a poor or a good job:

1. Do you know in your core that you did a good job? Could you have done better? If you could have done better, then take down notes on what you could have done and what you can do the next time. This will get your thoughts in order. Then admit that your boss has a reason to be dissatisfied. But don't beat yourself up. People make mistakes. Pick yourself up and try not to make that mistake again. If you have a good boss then just tell him you made a mistake and it won't happen again. If you have a great boss, you could outline your thoughts on how to improve your performance and get his thoughts as well. It will show to both yourself and your boss that you are in charge, you trust yourself, and you want to improve. If you have an idiot boss but he was right, just write down your notes for yourself, and work to improve your performance for your own satisfaction. Let me clarify that you shouldn't improve

yourself for others; you should do it for yourself alone, but getting people you trust to help you in the process is a great thing.

2. If you did a great job based on the parameters that you were given, then you are dealing with an insecure boss. He wanted something else but did not clarify that with you. Maybe he is getting a hard time from his boss and he turns around and takes it out on you. Don't let his issues affect you. In the first chapter, I mentioned that most people have issues and problems, and when they take it out on you, it is a reflection of them and not you. Well, this is a good example. The best way to quiet down your thoughts is to face the situation head on. Take some action. Talk to your boss instead of dragging the situation on for weeks. What a waste of time that would be. Speak to him; outline your position concerning how well you did your work and leave it at that. Your thoughts should be reinforced with phrases such as "I did my job," "I did it well based on the information or tools or people I had at my disposal," and "I am proud of myself." If the negative thoughts quiet down, it means you have solved the issue and you can move on. If the thoughts keep coming back and you are still daydreaming about the situation, then it is not resolved. You need to resolve it in order to move on. Go back to analyzing the situation; share the situation with someone who can put a new light on it. Face who or what you need to face to deal with it. If facing someone is not possible, write it all down in a letter and then burn the letter. Writing in your journal also helps. And do something physical. I cannot emphasize this enough. Get your body involved. Have a good work out and push yourself. It will help reunite your mind and body.

MORE ON RELATIONSHIPS WITH FOOD & BREAKING PATTERNS

It seemed that there was a relationship between events—all events—in my life and food. I wanted to celebrate a good thing: food. I felt anxious or stressed about a new project that was not going well: junk food. Someone made me feel like a nobody: more junk food. When I chose to binge when someone hurt my feelings, it was because at that specific moment I associated more pain to feeling that hurt then to breaking my promise to eat only healthy foods and maintain my weight. Did I feel better after? God, no. I felt the sting of the immediate pain less, but then felt disappointed with myself. I didn't feel love towards myself after a binging session, and I soon had a major stomachache, too.

What is so bad about feeling pain anyway? Why do we avoid it so much? The times when I succeeded at not throwing myself into binging and going through the pain, it was never that bad. I actually felt good that I was taking the time to listen to myself instead of avoiding or ignoring what was really going on. Imagine how you felt when someone you loved dismissed or ignored your pain. You do it to yourself every time you binge. I now find that the pain of not respecting my promise and the pain of seeing my goal of a healthy relationship towards food getting farther and farther away from me are a lot more painful than any immediate pain or anxiety I might feel. And that was an aha! moment. When I binged, the anxiety was reduced—yes, agreed—but the pain of trying to get back on track could last days, even weeks. And this feeling of disappointment would occur every time. That was my pattern: to alleviate my anxiety with food. Why did I develop this pattern and not another one? Who knows exactly, the mind is a funny thing. But I know it developed in my youth when food was used as a reward. It may also stem from the fact that we weren't rich when I was young, and we often wondered if we would have enough food, so the feeling of an empty stomach causes great anxiety for me.

Any of these feelings—loneliness, stress, rejection, empty stomach—makes me anxious. And feeling anxious makes me reach for food I should not have, and I eat and eat until I feel so full that the original pain disappears. Some people have said to me that I eat to fill a void. Feeling inadequate and feeling that my career is going nowhere are two indicators that I have a void to fill. But these two things give me extreme and repeated anxiety, which means they both need to be looked at more closely and I need to start resolving them one at a time. The answer was not only to break the pattern, but also to create a healthier pattern to deal with anxiety. To do this, I needed to spend time analyzing why I felt anxious in the first place.

One of the triggers for my pattern came from feeling rejected. It might come from my spouse or from someone at work or friends or family. It didn't matter. The feeling of rejection would turn into extreme anxiety and I could feel my stomach begin to churn.

First, I acknowledge the feeling. It is very easy for me because the minute that my body, mind, and soul want three chocolate bars and a bag of cookies, and chips that means something is wrong. So, I am thankful for that. I know something occurred to make me unhappy. Sometimes I need to go back a few hours or even a couple of days to figure out what, but usually, if I take the time to sit down and listen to myself, I will find out. Even if I didn't have those cravings, my daydreaming gives me good clues. If I daydream about being a victim or about being mean to someone, it usually means I am feeling hurt.

Second, I take action. Sometimes what occurred needs to be dealt with head on. I cannot ignore it (and God knows I have tried). Every time I did not confront someone that I felt had not treated me well, I got anxious, ate junk food, and then got angry. I am a sensitive person, so my threshold for feeling rejected is pretty low. I have to work on that and I am. Having said that, I now know that it is okay to speak to someone who hurt you and explain the situation. It is important that the discussion come from a place of caring for yourself and not a place of anger for the other person because you don't know how the other person will react so that is very important. If you let them know how they made you feel, most of the time you'll discover it was a misunderstanding or a miscommunication. In these days of emails and texting, the feeling behind the text does not always come through properly; a communiqué can sometimes be perceived as harsh when it was not meant to be. Because I write short and simple emails, people sometimes ask me if I am mad. I am not. I just like to get to the point.

Clearing the air is the key idea here. Don't forget that all people come into a room carrying their own stress and baggage and emotions and information they want to share. No matter how much they care (or not) for you, their lives come first to them and that is where their focus is. You will notice very few people pay attention to what you find so important (like losing 25 pounds!). Sorry but that is life. So don't be afraid to take some action. Speak to the person, write a letter, write in your journal, or go for walk and think it over. Do something that is positive for you. You don't have to make a big deal out of every situation, either. If you approach the person, then say you piece over coffee and move on. It's not a big deal to talk, but it is a big deal to respect your feelings, and that feels good. And don't wait to take action, the situation builds up and you become aggressive.

More often than not, a quick conversation will be sufficient. I know that my anxiety level will lower immediately, and I will resume my healthy eating habits. However, the other person may become nasty towards you and attack you. If this happens then, obviously, they are the problem, not you. Excuse the language coming up, but when this happens, say to yourself "Oh, ok, so you're an ass! That explains everything" and then stay away from them. This is easier said than done when that person is a sibling, a boss, a colleague, or a fellow student. But do your best. You cannot get rid of all the idiots around you; you can only control how you react to them. Take heart that once you become stronger, they will find another victim to attack. Until then, cut down, if possible, on the time you spend with them. I had to take some drastic measures in my personal life to ensure that only good people were in my close environment.

The key is to take action and do it now. And keep your eyes on the horizon and on your goals but not at the expense of ignoring current problems. You need to see both. Sometimes day-to-day life is not pleasant, and you need to keep visualizing your dreams and taking steps towards them every day. Working to find resolutions to these day-to-day problems will certainly help you attain your goals and dreams.

The way you act every day is a choice that you make, and you can choose to act differently. We often label ourselves, and come to believe certain things about ourselves (which is also a belief). Well that is how I labeled myself: I am an emotional eater and an all-or-nothing kind of girl. A few years ago, my dad said, "Why do you want to bother going to college? You are not that smart. Why don't you just get married and have kids?" As Oprah would say, I had an aha! moment. It was not right away or even conscious. I was upset and sad for many years that my father had such a low opinion of me. In time, I walked away from him and detached myself. I did finish college. I went on to university to get my bachelor's degree and then got my master's degree. But in the process, I had to walk away from someone because he did not elevate me but brought me down. It was hard but necessary because having a parent who thought this of me did not improve my self-esteem and kept the negative patterns in my life going.

Because of my dad's lack of confidence in me, I always felt that I was under the gun to perform. No one put pressure on me more than I put on myself. I always felt like I had to understand things the first time, and I had to do things well and quickly. And I always had to have a positive attitude. What unrealistic expectations I had for myself! That was the story I made for myself. So as soon as I felt criticized by others or by my own self, I felt unloved and started to look for junk food.

Now that we understand where behaviors and patterns come from, let's break them.

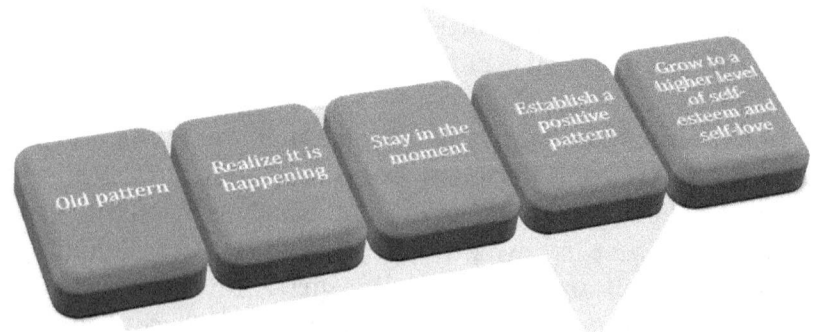

The best way to not let your younger self take over is to stay in the moment—in the present. This is the reality principle. Your reality today is not at all like your reality when you were younger. Things are different; you may now have your own salary, your own house, and your own children. You are free to leave if a situation is damaging your health or safety. Your life now is entirely different than when you were a child and were stuck living in your parents' house.

Here is how to get rid of a pattern:

Step 1: Identify the bad pattern.

Step 2: Link as much pain as possible to keeping that pattern. Visualize and feel all the very bad things that could happen to you if you were to keep that pattern for years. Think of all the great things you would miss out on, and feel the physiology of feeling down, sad, and depressed about missing out on these great things.

Step 3: Find a healthy pattern to replace the bad pattern. Link a great amount of pleasure to this new pattern, and visualize how amazing it will make you feel and how you'll feel years from now. Feel how amazing your life will turn out because you are going to change this simple pattern. Use your body physiology to reflect the new you.

Step 4: Re-create, in your head, the whole event that is causing you pain and visualize the new pattern. See how well you are doing, and link good feelings to the new pattern.

Repeat these steps until the new pattern feel like part of you—the new you, your new story. Choose your words carefully. Saying something is impossible is quite different than saying something is challenging but feasible.

For more details on how to perform these steps, I refer you to Tony Robbins'[4] CDs, which are amazing.

---

[4] Tony Robbins: Personal Power.

Staying in the present and staying focused is important. Once, I was writing in my journal and part of me wanted to stop writing and turn on the TV to OWN. Well, even if the OWN show I was going to watch would be helpful (*Finding Sarah*), I realized that it would be a diversion from what I was doing. And that was a red flag for me. Bells were ringing! I felt that if I kept writing I'd find something important, and I did. There was a huge cry for help from a hurt part of myself that was speaking to me, and, thank God I listened and did not try to cover it with TV or junk food. It was liberating.

Staying focused is challenging, but it gets easier. It is like a muscle: the more you use it, the stronger it becomes. Yes, the challenges get bigger as you grow, but you will be stronger and better equipped to handle them. When uncovering unknown youth pain, you never know what will come out. Sometimes it is something that is not so terrible, and you may tell yourself, "Wow, sweetie. I can deal with this. You did not have to suffer all this time over something that was not that dramatic." (Although it was dramatic to an eight year old, it may not be to a 40-something year old). Other times, you may uncover something that makes you feel uneasy, insecure, a little depressed, or weird. But so far, I have yet to uncover something that was such a bomb that I would have preferred not to remember. It all needs to come out, and your younger self, who remembers, needs to know that it is okay to come out. That younger self needs to know that you will be there with love and respect no matter what. Don't forget that if you feel the need to see a therapist, it is okay. Do not hesitate; it will help you get closer to your goals.

Now that patterns have been looked at, it is important to talk about beliefs. Both are important foundation stones for the perceptions we have of ourselves.

BELIEFS

Now, what is a belief? According to Wikipedia, ***Belief*** *is the psychological state in which an individual holds a proposition or premise to be true.*

For example, I believe that I need to struggle to keep the weight off. I also believe that I can take the weight off, but I don't believe I can keep it off forever. I also believe that I will run out of food. I have to eat as much as I can in a given meal; I cannot leave anything on my plate in case there is no food at the next meal. So I believe that I need to have a full stomach all the time to make sure I am okay.

So how do you change an unhealthy belief? By replacing it with a new and healthy one. A healthy belief is a belief that is good for you and helps you grow into the person you want to be. The best way to read about how to do this is with Tony Robbins' audio CDs[5]. The first time I heard them, I was not quite ready to absorb everything he said, but time and again I refer to them to solve specific things. I would also like to refer you to Jack Canfield's book about this as his method worked for me.[6]

When you work at replacing a belief, adding lots of emotions and feelings to the beliefs will help the process work much better. I want to remove pain from my life and add joy, so I need to reduce the pain of the old beliefs and make fun of them. These two combinations will make the process work faster. Remember that beliefs that are linked to your younger years took such a hold because they came out of deep, strong emotions.

---

[5] Tony Robbins: Personal Power
[6] Jack Canfield: The Success Principles: how to get from where you are to where you want to be.

How to Remove a Limiting Belief:

Step 1: Name your limiting belief. In my case, it was the belief that I wouldn't always have enough food to eat. The feelings behind this belief were feeling scared and insecure, and anxious about starving.

Step 2: Make fun of the belief in a positive way to remove the stigma of pain. For me, I repeated my visualization out loud multiple times.

"I live in a land where everything is made out of good healthy food and some chocolate. I dance, sing, and play with the food. It will never go or disappear. It is always there for me. While I am dancing, I am dressed like Katy Perry—all in food."

The last image is silly, but it makes me smile when I visualize it.

Step 3: Create a new belief, a healthy one.
There is plenty of amazing food for me anytime I want it.

According to Jack Canfield,[7] you have to repeat your new belief multiple times a day, for a minimum of 30 days. Some beliefs were so hard to kick for me that I had to say them for up to two or sometimes three months. It works faster if you are 100% committed and have tons of great feelings about the new belief. What I do is keep a small booklet in my purse, and every time a belief pops into my head, I write it down and then I do this exercise. I only do one belief at a time. When I have moved on from a belief, I go to my booklet and I pick and choose the next one that bothers me the most. Visualizing your life with this new belief is also a great help.

---

[7] Jack Canfield: The Success Principles: how to get from where you are to where you want to be.

Perception is a dangerous thing. How you perceive a situation, how you perceive yourself or others can make or break you. I developed a perception of myself based on what adults told me when I was young, and I am still working at changing those bad perceptions. It is not always easy, but it is worth it. I have had to remove the stigma and bad emotions of my past, and I've done that by linking them to a simple pattern and changing the pattern. When you play the victim, and when you say you are who you are because of what happened 30 years ago, it can get difficult. So take one thing at a time. Confirm if it is a belief or a pattern and then change it. Add great feelings to the new pattern and belief; visualize all the good that this new perception is going to bring into your life. Believe you are fully responsible for your life and actions and stop blaming everyone else or any past event. Act as if right now that you are living with the new belief or pattern.

Isn't it amazing how many years we can carry unnecessary burdens? Don't you deserve a better life? Does that person who hurt you really deserve all that time you are giving them? It is time. There is plenty of help out there to help you find freedom to become the best you. Take it one day at a time. You did not become who you are in one day. But the more you work on yourself, the better you will feel, and the more you will want to do and the faster the process will go. It does not have to be painful. I have broken some established patterns, including smoking, and I am amazed at how easy they were to break. Once you are ready in your mind, heart, and soul, once you are committed 100% to getting it done, it is a piece of cake!

Chapter 2 Summaries

- ➢ Take 100% responsibility for your life, choices, and actions.
- ➢ Identify your bad patterns and change them for great ones that help you grow.
- ➢ Associate feelings with your old and new patterns.
- ➢ Identify your bad beliefs and change them for great ones that help you grow.
- ➢ Is your perception of a situation accurate? Spend time reviewing it, without affects.
- ➢ Rewrite your story how you want it to be. Don't let old stories define who you are today.

Chapter 3: Control Your Thoughts

All that is necessary to break the spell of inertia and frustration is this: Act as if it were impossible to fail.

DOROTHEA BRANDE
A well-respected writer and editor

If you read only one chapter or remember only one chapter, this is the one. This one will change your life. Your thoughts really are the beginning of who you will be tomorrow. What you thought yesterday, last week, last month makes you who you are today. I used to think, "I need to struggle to keep my weight off," and that was who I was. Isn't that amazing?

Before we go further, I want to emphasize that I don't know what your personal situation is. If you have deep psychological problems, I trust you are seeing a specialist. There are many fantastic therapies out there, and there is one that is right for you. You have to believe in your core that you deserve an amazing life and sometimes you need a specialist to help you get rid of old traumas that are lingering.

OTHER PEOPLE'S THOUGHTS

One of the hardest perceptions for me to change was my view of my physical self after I lost the weight. I had lost 25 pounds, I had done multiple treatments to help with cellulite, and the before and after pictures were amazing. I was eager to try on bathing suits for my honeymoon. I had arrived, but instead of thinking, "Wow! I look amazing!" I was focusing on the flaws. I had exactly the same speech in my head as I had before I lost the weight. My solution? Lose another 10 pounds! Brilliant! But would I accept myself after I'd lost an additional 10 pounds? No. I can tell you, I would not feel better about myself even if I lost another 10 more pounds. I needed to drastically change my perception of myself and more specifically, my thoughts.

Many people have told me that they find me beautiful, and some tell me that I look easily 10 years younger than I am, but I feel like they there are talking about someone else. I did not relate to what they were saying. *That's not me!* Then I realized that this speech in my head was the speech of my teenage self when I was perceived by others as an ugly duck compared to my sister (and she pounded me with that perception, too!). Boy was I tired of carrying around voices from 30 years ago. It helped to think about where those nasty thoughts and voices came from. Knowing it came from mostly siblings who were insecure about themselves and brought me down to raise themselves up shone a new light on things. I was at the point where I wanted to give those thoughts back to them! You can keep 'em! I am beautiful, and I look young because I am crazy about facials and non-surgical treatments like redness reduction, skin tightening, and a disciplined face-cleansing regimen. I am also crazy about cellulite treatments, creams, and massages. I work out regularly, I eat healthy, and I restrict dessert, alcohol, and bad carbs. That is why I look good, and that is why I am proud when my husband tells me I look amazing.

Everyone has thousands and thousands of thoughts per day. I am not asking you to monitor them all. That would be a full-time job. But you can monitor the dominant ones. It is not easy. When you have been doing something for ten or twenty years you can't change it overnight. So how do we do it?

Chapter 3: Control Your Thoughts

Step 1: For three full days, monitor your thoughts[8] Include one day off in there (one week-end day). And really do it. Write down or record everything that passes through your head. It is arduous, but it is necessary to be able to move on to the next step. As the saying goes, how do you know where you're going if you don't know where you are! Where you are, is who you are today with your current thoughts and the thoughts of the past months and years. So go on and log them. My therapist thought writing down everything might be dangerous because it might put me in a depressive mood to discover all the negative thoughts in my head. My thinking, however, was that it was already there and it was affecting my life negatively, so why not face it? So I did. And I still do.

Step 2: The next step is to replace those thoughts. But how do you get rid of a thought? Replace it with another one, a stronger one. Don't just mumble your new thought; attach positive and strong emotions to it.

Let's do an example:

I used to wake up and anything and everything that could happen to me during the day, I perceived in a negative way. Whether it was a meeting, an encounter with someone I did not particularly like, or the numbers of things that could or would go wrong during events happening that day. I imagined all the bad things that could happen. When I started logging my thoughts, I could not believe how many negative thoughts I had going on in there, totally unmonitored. No wonder I went through life anxious all the time: I was living with negativity day in and day out! The thing is, I knew I could manage those thoughts and have an amazing, relaxing day. Do you remember the last time you had one of those? Do you

---

[8] Jack Canfield: The Success Principles: how to get from where you are to where you want to be.

remember waking up feeling amazing and having that feeling last all day? Do you remember when you were relaxed, people were relaxed around you, and everything went the right way? Why not aim at living every day like that!

THOUGHTS TO LISTEN TO

One note about the difference between a negative thought and a warning thought: You need to be able to differentiate between the two and pay attention to the latter. Let's say, for example, you need to go in front of a board of directors to ask and get approval on financing for a special project. You prepare everything and when you practice your speech, you have those annoying voices that tell you this or that might go wrong, or that you have to prepare your answers in case someone in the group does not agree with your points. Play the devil's advocate, and go ahead and prepare answers to the worst possible objections or questions you can imagine. It is basic preparation. Those thoughts are ok since they help you be more ready for a big event.

Monitoring your thoughts so they are rewarding instead of punishing does not mean you shouldn't listen to your intuition. You have to listen to your intuition at all times because it can be useful. But, if a thought that is not rewarding or not helping you reach your goal keeps coming back, it may be worthwhile to pounder it a bit. Don't be mechanical in changing your thoughts, although for some of them you can be mechanical. For little things, for example, such as "I will miss the bus and get all upset." You can change it for, "I will be smart and organize appropriately and leave early and take a peaceful walk to the bus instead of rushing to catch the bus."

HOW DID I DO IT?

After three days of logging all my negative thoughts, I knew my pattern. And instead of waking up feeling negative about my day, I started to feel grateful. I'd lie in bed a bit longer and I'd go through everything I enjoyed about my life: my husband, my health, a good paying job, nice colleagues and friends, etc. This set the tone for the day. Then I got up and worked out most days, and then I'd meditate. At the end of my meditation, I spent some time visualizing my day. If I had to do something I didn't like that day, I'd put a positive spin on it. I'd visualize myself as calm, relaxed, and centered throughout the day. This is exactly what I did when I visualized my wedding. I did not allow any negative thoughts to enter. Negative thoughts are like weeds: if you let one in, more and more will grow. Every time I had a negative thought, I replaced it consciously with a positive one and attached feelings to the new thought. I cannot emphasize enough how important it is to add feelings (joy, happiness, contentment, satisfaction, etc.) to your new thought. At first, it is a process that will require a lot of focus. I found that when I did something habitual like brushing my teeth, I had to focus more and not let my mind wander. I wanted to use that time to improve my well-being. More and more the new thinking pattern became a habit. Now, the days that I get up and don't do what I have outlined here, I don't feel as good and my day is most definitely not as rewarding.

If you ever wonder if a thought is good or bad, here's a test. Imagine yourself saying that thought to your daughter, son, best friend, or your partner. Would you say it? Or, would you say something nicer, more rewarding, and more positive? If the answer is yes, then don't you think you deserve the same? YES, you do.

SMILE

Smile. When you are just having a bad day, push your shoulders back, take a deep breath, and smile even if you don't feel like it. I had read that but never quite understood how a smile could impact your mood until I started doing it on a regular basis. Natalie Cole sings a song "Smile." I love that song. When I am feeling down or my mind wants to keep focusing on bad things, I listen to it and I do it—I smile.

I also like to remind myself that what is making me sad or mad or anxious today will mean nothing in a week, a month, or a year. I say the phrase, "This too shall pass." Most things are not worth me losing my calm, my happiness, and my joy.

Eventually, the negative thoughts will disappear.

WHAT DO I DO EXACTLY?

On a day-to-day basis, what does all this mean?

1. Log your negative thoughts for three days.
2. Replace negative thoughts with positive ones and feel them.
   a. I am a success
   b. I am a winner
   c. I am a kind person
   d. I am successfully achieving this goal
   e. I deserve wealth

3. Your old self will fight this all it can, but speak kindly to yourself and tell yourself that you are ready to move on. In fact, act as if you have already achieved your goal. When you visualize, look at yourself having

succeeded in six months, one year, five years, 10 years, and 20 years. It will help you focus your thoughts.

4. What helps me is looking at myself in the mirror. When my little voice is screaming with fear and anxiety, it calms me to look at myself. I am not an eight year old but a forty-something year old who is in control. Look into your eyes. Let the emotions come up if they are ready. Don't stop them from coming out, use it as an opportunity to manage them. But don't force them. Sometimes I find they are not ready, and my younger one just quiets down.

5. Exercise discipline. Your old self will try everything to get you to do things the old way, to stay in the comfort zone. Just say no. Do not leave any doors open.

6. Open your heart. What I mean by that is, be open to good things happening in your life. I know why none of the things I wanted happened earlier: I was not ready to receive them. When I started putting into practice the things I mention here, one day very early on, I got a call from a publishing consulting firm. Would you believe that my reaction was frustration that the publisher was disturbing me at my work? Why couldn't they write me or send me the information through email so I could read it when I had time? And that happened on a slow day. The Universe was answering my prayer to become a published author, and I refused to see it and welcome it. I wonder how many of these I refused to see or never even noticed. Open your heart. Believe it can happen. By the way, I called back the publisher the same day and got all kinds of great information.

7. This step is very important: act *as-if.* If your old self and your old thoughts brought you to where you are today, imagine where you want to be and start thinking and acting as if you were there already. My husband and I got fed up, seriously fed up, with the harsh winters in Canada. We love San Diego, and we try to go there every year on vacation. One year I said that we should look at condos there even if we were not ready to move there yet. And I wanted to look at high-end condos as if we could afford it. I explained to him the concept of acting *as-if.* It is a great tool for everything you want to accomplish in your life. It also helps to establish if you are heading in the right direction. You know you are heading in the right direction when it feels good. We are so good at hiding how we feel with food and alcohol that we don't recognize how we feel anymore. Imagine you have this dream of being a boss, a leader. You start acting *as-if,* you start dressing like an executive, you start taking your place and speaking up at meetings. You start helping and coaching people but then realize that you are getting increasingly uncomfortable. You realize that maybe leading people is not for you; maybe your focus should be to excel and be the best at something else. Look deeper and work at identifying your talent and start developing it and be the best at that instead. Listen and feel. Your body, your heart, and your soul have all the answers for you. You just have to listen.

These are the tricks that I have used to help me change my thoughts. The old me still peeps up every once in a while, don't get me wrong. It takes consistent focus for a long time to settle into your real self and let go of all those layers of faux self that got added on to you through the different experiences you went through in life and through the different people you met.

Chapter 3: Control Your Thoughts

It is important to emphasize that nothing will change unless you change your thoughts. I notice that I have a harder time focusing on good and positive thoughts when I am tired or sick. This is when mantras are useful. Keep your mantra positive, powerful, and simple. It is better to repeat a mantra then to let your mind wander in places you don't want it to go.

IDEAS

Instead of	Replace with
I don't like my thighs, stomach, etc.	I love my smile, my hair, my eyes, etc.
This meeting will be hell	I will learn XX at this meeting. I will see XX that I like.
I hate my job	I like that I am able to pay for things I want and need. I made a few of good friends through work. And I met my husband at work! It is good that I am dissatisfied, now I can look at what I want and change. Tony Robbins says that being dissatisfied is the best state to be in: it gets you moving.
I can't stand that person	Focus on people you like and enjoy. Don't give any space in your mind to those people you don't like. Don't let them live rent-free in your head!
I won't be able to keep the weight off	That is an old voice and belief from years past. Good-bye! Who I am today is a woman who loves to be healthy and happy with her food and exercise choices. My resolve, my strength, my courage and my persistence help me make the right

	food choices and exercise choices every day in order to optimize my health.

Have fun with change. Make fun of your negative thoughts and sometimes change them with a joke. It removes the feeling of drama that often accompanies negative thoughts." Also, use your affirmations—positive, rewarding, and with great feelings—to replace lingering negative thoughts.

HOW LONG?

You probably want to know how long it will take. The only possible answer is "as long as it needs to." It depends on how strong or thick the wall is; the one you are tearing down. How long did it take you to be where you are today? How ready are you to make a change? At the very least, it will take consistent daily efforts for months for your negative thoughts to change into positive, rewarding ones. You will run into roadblocks and serious resistance. You will encounter your own obstacles and life's obstacles as well. Just keep in mind that life's roadblocks or obstacles are tests. They will test you to see if you are ready to move on to the next stage. Just by knowing that, your attitude towards them should change. You should welcome them and scream out loud, "Yes! I am ready for them. I am ready to get through them and move on to my higher self." If you don't face your obstacles, they will keep coming back until you do. I am a firm believer that they show up when we are ready to deal with them. Keep in mind that you cannot grow if you don't go through these events. If you think you have solved a negative aspect of yourself that you wanted to get rid of, I can guarantee life will test you to make sure you have.

Chapter 3: Control Your Thoughts

Maria Angelou wrote that words are things.[9] Well, your thoughts are things, too. They are real: they create your life. I was literally at a crossroads. I knew I had to change my thoughts if I wanted my life to change. By some standards, I had already managed to succeed in my life. I had come from a poor family to take two major degrees and become vice-president of a major IT consulting firm. And most importantly, having attracted in my life the most amazing, gorgeous man who is kind, funny, hugely smart, and loving. So I must have done something right! But somewhere in me, there were old voices that stated that I did not believe I deserved any of it. It all belonged to someone else, and it was just a matter of time before I lost it all, self-sabotage you know. It took me 20 years to achieve everything I had and those were my thoughts. Imagine! It had been so hard and painful to achieve, but I had managed it because somewhere I believed in me and I invested in long-term psychoanalytical therapy. But only recently, with the help of that therapy, did I start believing I deserved what I had. I still had the odd thought that I did not deserve it, but by controlling my thoughts and reinforcing my belief in myself those thoughts were fewer and farther between.

I didn't want to take another 20 years to get a point where I 100% believed that I deserved it. This was when I realized that I had to completely and irrevocably change how I perceived myself. And it started with my thoughts. Out with the old and in with the new.

TEST

One day I got my test. I was having a relaxing day off from work, and when I was plagued by negative thinking (it did not

---

[9] I heard that on OWN, Masters' show.

matter if it was a day of work or a day off, I could find negative things to complain about), I told myself that I had resolved all that so I was relaxed. Then things happened to me over two days that were unbelievable. I had an appointment at the bank for a new account. The manager was sick and she rescheduled for the next day. I had hurt my neck and needed to see my osteopath, but she was also sick and had to reschedule. I spent all Labor Day weekend in pain. When we did get to the bank, my husband and I opened a new account, but there were problems with the computer, and we were there two hours instead of the planned thirty minutes. The bank told us that by later that night we'd have online access to our account. That night my husband got online, but it took two days before I could access the account. I had outstanding checks but could not deposit money into the account! Earlier in the week, my husband and I had gone to an office supply store to buy some office furniture and have them delivered. It is one of those places that say between 9 and 5. They cannot tell you a specific hour. So we wasted one day of not planning anything on our mini-vacation waiting for the furniture to arrive. It arrived early but—surprise, surprise—that was only piece number one. They did not deliver everything at once! We waited again, and the second deliveryman finally came and then suggested I go downstairs to the front door to get the furniture myself! I said, I don't think so!" So he brought it upstairs. After he'd gone, as my husband and I opened the box, we realized it was the wrong size. It was not what we ordered. I called the store and they confirmed it was the wrong size. They asked me to wait yet another full day for the exchange. By then I had started to voice my frustration, but my husband has a saying: "He who loses control, loses." So I tried to return to my calm self and the store agreed to a delivery window of between nine and noon on Saturday for the exchange. Later that day, my husband had some business to attend to, so I decided to go downtown to relax and shop. He was going to join me later for drinks. I was standing in front of the cashier at the first store when I realized I had forgotten my wallet at home. I remembered that I had taken out my wallet to try that new bankcard yet again and I had never put the wallet back in my purse. At this point, it was all so absurd that I started laughing right there at the counter. The events of those two days were ridiculous, and I had to walk back home because I had no money for a cab. During all these events, I kept telling myself two things. One: It is a test to see if you are really able to not freak out when something does not go your way. Two: In a week from now, you won't remember these two days, so is it really worth losing your calm?

I am very proud to say I did not lose my calm. And because I had come home to get my wallet, I was there when my husband returned, so we were able to go shopping together and then go relax at our favorite bar. It ended up being a very nice few hours together. And my osteopath called and was able to fit me in the same week, so all that was taken care of. People who saw the positive side of things used to annoy me. Now I have joined their ranks and proudly. It is amazing the free time you find when you stop complaining about everything and instead focus on what is good out there.

In this chapter, you have some tricks to get you going. I also suggest you review other readings at the end of the book. What amazes me is that I have succeeded in life despite recurring negative thoughts. But those thoughts were starting to weigh heavier than ever on me. I really wanted them gone and I didn't want to be split in two all the time. I want all my selves to go into one direction; I want to be one, a strong core. I look at pictures of me as a kid and I see that I actually was gorgeous. If I had lived in a nurturing environment, God knows how different my life could have been. Well, as an adult, I have the power to change all that. That is the power of thoughts, the power of words, and, therefore, the power of who I become. I can change, one slow moment at a time. I don't think there are any magic tricks. You might try hypnosis, if you believe in it, but, personally, I think the process is so much more important than the result. The idea is to reconnect with your self and to heal. No quick fix solution can do that. You need to do it yourself; no healer or therapist can do that for you. They can only guide you. My point is, you only need you. You have the power to rediscover love for yourself. You lost it a while back and that is okay. You are where you are now; just go from there.

Don't look for love outside of you. (Easier said than done when your entire life you have looked outside for validation as I have.) Don't look for it in your mom, dad, siblings, friends, or life partner. If your thoughts are negative and hurtful towards your own self, then you need to find the love in your own self. Go where the problem is. Don't try to cover it up. The love is there. It was always there under layers of hurtful thoughts and words, your own and others. Now you know why this step is important. It is a crucial period. You are against a brick wall and that brick wall prevents you from reaching the self-love that's on the other side. Get rid of that darn wall. (The wall is you, by the way, in case you did not get that.) It's time. One thought at a time, one hour at a time, and one day at time. Change your thoughts for positive and self-rewarding ones, and the bricks will fall one at a time.

Chapter 3 Summaries

➢ List your bad thoughts for three days, including one "off" day.
➢ Change those negative thoughts for positive ones.
➢ Smile and "fake it until you make it."
➢ Relearn to love yourself and be kind to yourself.
➢ Keep an eye out for tests and challenges that will help you grow.

Chapter 4: Write in Your Journal

The act of putting pen to paper encourages pause for thought, this in turn makes us think more deeply about life, which helps us regain our equilibrium.

NORBERT PLATT
CEO of Rollei Singapore and Managing Director
of Rollei Fototechnic in Germany

The theme of this book is the rediscovery of your self, your true self. To open communication with your core being. Writing in your journal will help accomplish that. In the age of iPods and intelligent phones, it seems we are connected with everyone and everything, but really not with ourselves, so I suggest writing in your journal, every day if possible. Some suggest writing first thing in the morning while some suggest writing at night before bedtime as a way to recap the day. I say follow what feels right for you. I have tried to do it at night without much success. For me the morning works best. I am usually half-asleep and have no blockage. I write everything that comes to mind. In fact, that is how the idea of this book came about. That is when I have most of my big revelations. I do suggest writing by hand and not on the computer. You want to remove all electronics from this exercise. Go back to basics. Treat yourself to a great fountain pen and writing material. If you want more information on this, I recommend you read *The Artist's Way* by Julia Cameron. It is an amazing book.

Are there any guidelines to write in your journal? Not really. But here are some ideas to get you going.

1. You can recap the day before. Write about what you felt went right or wrong, why and how to improve. For

example, one of the exercises in the early chapters is to stop thinking negative thoughts. You could recap that. Did you have some? At what particular time? Did you replace them with good thoughts? Why or why not? How could you improve? I know this is a little mechanical, but it is useful if you want to improve or get rid of bad habits.

2. How do you want the day ahead of you to go? It is becoming general knowledge that if you see your day developing a certain way, there is a big chance that it will happen exactly as you saw and felt it. It helps to outline what kind of day you want to have and how to make it happen. You view your whole day—meetings, people you will see—and you decide how you will react to those events. Will you be relaxed and happy or stressed and anxious? As you know, you cannot control outside events, but you can control how you react to those events. I find that the days I plan ahead tend to go the way I planned. When I am overwhelmed and I don't do this, the day tends to go a little less smoothly. I did that for my wedding. I was determined to have a day where I was going to enjoy myself, where I was going to be relaxed, and where there was going to be no major glitch. It worked. It was perfect.

3. Write about feelings you're experiencing towards yourself or someone else or towards a situation. The situation may be, for example your job. Are you happy with your job? Do you feel fulfilled by it? Is there anything you can do to improve it? You might also write about feelings towards someone who is currently in your life or no longer in your life. Sometimes you need to clear out old things you are still carrying. I am tired of carrying the habit of negative and persecution thoughts that got started 30 years ago in my home life.

I was still carrying grudges against people after all these years. If it is necessary to clean up your past, writing in your diary can help identify people or grudges that you need to address. You might also try the exercise of writing a letter to a specific person. It can include how you were feeling in the past, how you are feeling now, and how their behavior hurt you. You can mail it or you can burn it, but you have to write it from a place of forgiveness.

4. Sometimes you will feel that you have a blockage or have nothing to say, nothing is coming out. If this happens, then recap your day or plan the next day. Or, you can try an exercise from this book or other books. Some exercises I've used include making lists: list all your successes by age—0 to 15, 15 to 30, 30 to 45, etc.; or list all the things you want in life—the material things, the talents you want to develop, the job you want, the friends you want, the spouse you want, the places you want to live in or visit. Sometimes, I play *as-if* in my journal: if you're in the middle of the year, pretend it is December 31st and write down how the rest of the year panned out. It is fun and it puts everything in a new light.

I have noticed that sometimes writing can be mechanical for the first 15 or 20 minutes. Then I seem to enter a deeper level of myself and things come out. These things may be related to the topic I am writing about but not always. It is important to pay attention to your thoughts when you go through this exercise. Log your thoughts as they pop up. It may mean you need to focus on something else right now.

A lot of the aha! moments I have had in my life came while I was writing in my journal. I find it a simple tool but worth the trouble. It opens gates of communications. It is amazing. Try it once in a while at first to see how it feels. Do longer sessions on your days off. I think you'll find it beneficial. Every once in a while, review your progress. At the end of the year, you could spend time reviewing the past year and establishing goals for the next year. I don't wait until the end of the year anymore, now I review every quarter. It is easier to remember the past three months than the past 12. Give it a try. It is some alone time that you well deserve. If you feel that once a day is too much, start with 2-3 times a week.

Chapter 4 Summaries

> ➤ Morning or night, take some time off for yourself and write in your journal.
> ➤ Write by hand. Treat yourself to a nice pen and a wonderful journal.
> ➤ Indulge in longer sessions on your days off.
> ➤ From time to time, review your progress. Go back and read what you have written.

Chapter 5: Imagine Your Future and Act *As-If*

*For time and the world do not stand still. Change is the law of life.
And those who look only to the past or the present are certain to miss
the future.*

JOHN F. KENNEDY
35th president of the United States of America

At the beginning of this book, I wrote that we were disappointed because we had imagined all kinds of good things happening once we'd lost the weight. For me, however, nothing happened. You know why? Because I brought me along! The old me. I realized that I couldn't expect things to change if I was still the same inside. I still had to work on my thoughts. Not easy! I just had to keep persevering. There was and there is no way around it.

So yes, you have lost the pounds but nothing else has really changed, or barely. You are a little more active. You may be spending less time in front of the TV. You now take the time to prepare your food. You like shopping a little more. And those changes may affect some of the things or the people around you. Cause and effect. But you need to figure out what is disappointing you. Are you disappointed in the way you feel towards yourself or food? The fact that you did not get that modeling contract? The way people are around you? Log it all. In order to pinpoint where you're going, you have to know where you are, remember? It's important to log your feelings towards what you did not get, as well as make a list of what you expected. We need to manage those expectations. Ideally, you made that list before losing the weight and now you can compare. If you didn't make a list before you started, that's okay. I didn't either; it was pure raw emotion that made me lose the weight before my wedding.

So here is my written list after my weight loss of what I expected to happen:

1. I expected to finally feel calm. I expected to feel calm about my relationship with food, calm with myself (meaning happy and content with my body and the way I looked), and calm as a human being. I didn't want to always feel anxious about everything. (Wow, talk about managing expectations; I did not achieve that, obviously!)

2. I expected my relationships with others to be different. I expected everyone to marvel at my accomplishment. Then I expected to be treated like a goddess—treated with the utmost respect. I expected to be able to say, "How dare you speak to me this way! Now I am gorgeous and I succeeded in losing weight—something most people fail at—through a strong will and with courage. I am, therefore, above you! Oh, boy!

3. I expected to have an amazing wedding. I expected to fit into my dress perfectly. I expected the guests to freak out at how amazing I looked. And I expected to have fun and be relaxed.

4. I expected to get a modeling contract. Quite a few people mentioned how good I looked, so why not?

5. I expected to become rich. I didn't have any specifics on how this would happen, but I associate being thin with being rich.

6. In sum, I expected to be beautiful, not longer work in an IT firm, be a successful model, rich, and live somewhere warm and beautiful.

Now that I am writing this down, I say to myself, "Good God women! How old are you? Twelve?" These are not realistic expectations! But don't let this voice affect your list as you write it. Don't be logical when you make it. It has to come from deep inside of you. That is important because you need to manage your expectations, and if you do not list all the unrealistic ones, you won't deal with them.

So that's ok, one can dream, and if you're going to dream, dream BIG. I am usually a very logical and organized person, so these expectations came from a side of me that is younger and creative with a big imagination! Being who I am, I decided to look at each of these, to see what went wrong.

So I reviewed each of my expectations. And, of course, I suggest you do this exercise as well.

1. I expected to feel calm. I lost the weight in eight months. But I have been anxious for over 30 years. The anxiety was not going to disappear in eight months. I guess I associated my anxiety to being fat.

    I have spoken at length about my anxiety. I can offer one piece of advice: Everything you are and you feel has multiple levels. Because you wrote about it once, because you analyzed it once, because you spoke about it once to a friend, does not mean you have covered all the layers. Going over something twice or multiple times is not a bad thing. You may understand or assimilate something today that you did not yesterday. So if something keeps coming back to you, keep on reviewing it.

    I knew I had to spend a bit more time trying to understand why I was anxious all the time. My anxiety exists on multiple levels. My anxiety with food began at a very young age. Like many parents, they used food as a reward and punishment mechanism. Because we were not rich, what we had was limited and we were not able to have food whenever we wanted. Don't get me wrong: I never went one day without food. My parents did amazing things with little money. But if I was hungrier one day, I could not go in the fridge or pantry to get extra food. I sometimes did, but in secret. School lunches were not with those fancy drinks and desserts; they were just regular sandwiches and an apple. As a result, I was jealous of other kids. When the weather was good, I did love walking home for lunch when I could have a hot dog and fries—that was a treat. I grew up feeling scared that I would not have enough food. My parents spoke openly about their money problems in front of us. That created the belief in me that there might not be enough food. That resulted in binging. When I got my hands on food, I binged thinking I might not have enough food later. If I was punished as a child, I was sent to my room without dinner, which was horrible for a child and did not promote a very good night's sleep. This relationship with food continued into my college years when I had to fend for myself and I had very little money working as a waitress and studying. So that kind of relationship with food has been going on for a very long time. It was not going to disappear just because I lost 25 pounds or because I had more money. This was a major discovery for me. Another discovery was that because fancy desserts (chocolate bars, chips, gummy bears) were seldom seen in our home, every time I got my hands on one, I felt rich. That was a second belief I had about food, again not a healthy one: "To have fancy treats (junk food) meant I can afford them, which meant I was rich." I never realized I had that belief until I started writing things down.

2. My relationships with others did change, but not the way I thought they would. First of all, I was happier and smiled more. People react differently to you when you smile than when you are angry and moody. That reaction, however, has nothing to do with my weight. The second thing I noticed was the looks. After losing the weight, I started wearing nice office suits and skirts, and I think I walked

with more confidence. People react to that. I did get the oohs and ahs and "You look amazing!" comments, but they lasted only a couple of days. I couldn't expect them to last forever. It was clear that my expectations were very, very immature. It goes back to my need to be loved and my need for external validation. Also, keep in mind that people have their own lives to worry about. They don't spend that much time thinking about you.

3. The wedding. This one came through 150%. It was better than I could have ever imagined and the pictures prove it. I look happy and relaxed, laughing and smiling a lot at the pre-wedding preparations, the ceremony, and after. The dress fit amazingly well, and I looked fantastic. People commented on how amazing I looked. Everyone loved the wedding. My husband and I are so much in love and it showed. It was a love wedding, and we made sure to be surrounded with people we really cared for.

4. I expected to be given a modeling contract by simply walking down the street and being discovered. Well! Not so much! What I should have asked is why I wanted it or needed it? This question may help in attaining some, but do not forget that sometimes you do not get what you want because it is not your path. I wanted to model because I wanted more money in my life, and it seemed like an easy way to get it. I also thought that doing a full portfolio with a photographer and then showing it around would confirm to myself that I am a good-looking person. Yes, this is the need for external validation again. Yes I keep on working on my own self worth and looking less and less outside of myself for validation. I always felt like an ugly duck and I was becoming a swan and I wanted people to know it. Now that I have grown and learned a few things, I have decided that being a model is not what I want. I did do the portfolio and even had a magazine

printed out of it. And, it looks amazing, but I decided to do it for me. Only my husband and my best friend have seen it. It is private. I believe now that I am beautiful, and I don't have to be a model because I don't have to prove it to anyone.

5. Being thin does not equal being rich. Being thin naturally and in a healthy way means I have resolved some past issues that prevented me from moving forward. As those issues are resolved, I have the guts to do things that I did not before, such as writing this book. And that may help my finances. When I was younger, I wanted to be rich at whatever cost. Now being happy and fulfilled is more important than being rich. It would be nice to have more money to enjoy life with my husband, yes, because I firmly believe we deserve the first-class seats on the plane and the five-star hotels. But my choice of career is now based on being happy and fulfilled.

6. Leave the company I worked for. I expected this to happen right away. Things take time, but sometimes I wish they would go faster. I am not very patient. I read the following fable. A man saw a cocoon and decided to help the caterpillar become a butterfly, so he started removing layers of the caterpillar's cocoon to free the upcoming butterfly. Once he'd removed the protective shell, however, the butterfly emerged, tried to fly but fell down and died. The butterfly did not take the time for the journey and to get ready to be the beautiful butterfly he was going to become. That's why the journey is so important, and that's also why you have to fully trust that things happen when they're supposed to happen. Don't let anyone rush you into something if you don't feel ready. Trust your gut and your intuition. And be patient. I am my worst enemy in this regard. When I have realized or fixed something that was blocking me, I want things to change

right then and there. I have to be thin and I have to have my own business and it has to happen now. Relax and enjoy the journey. I have had years of hard work to get me ready to welcome it. It is that simple.

ACT *AS-IF*

What it all comes down to is this: Are you 100% committed? What is preventing you from acting as if you have already achieved a higher level of self-being and self-worth? Acting *as-if* says it all. I have spoken about this in an earlier chapter, but let's go into more detail here. For example, you want to be treated with respect. First, treat others with respect. Then act right now *as-if* you are not the type of person who tolerates being disrespected. If you want to have a great relationship with food, act *as-if* you have already achieved your goal. You know what needs to be done to get there. Fake it 'til you make it, as they say. You want a healthy body image? Act *as-if* you already have love for yourself and your body. Dress well; never leave the house feeling that you look horrible. Relaxed? Yes. Horrible? No. Treat yourself well now: do those home facials, take those baths, and sleep in on the weekends. If you have kids, make a deal with your spouse. One weekend he sleeps in and one weekend you do. Feel that you can say "no" when saying "yes" will make you unhappy. Don't wait until you feel you can do it: start now. Act *as-if* now. Start small and move up from there. It is all inside you for the taking. Just act *as-if* you are now the person you want to be. As soon as you say "soon," "someday," "next year," or "January 1st," you are saying "later." It never means now. Don't you want to feel that way now? Then do it. And at the same time, work with a specialist for deeper issues. Work at changing your patterns and beliefs, monitoring your thoughts, and saying those affirmations. All the techniques we have reviewed so far work.

They really do!

But they work only if you do them consistently. Don't forget that you have years of self-abuse to get rid of. You know what I had a hard time with? Confirming what my beliefs were. I had some kind of blockage. It took time but suddenly they came rushing out of my head. And they did while I was writing in my journal. The basic idea here is that you should not to wait until December 31st to see what worked and what did not throughout the year. You want to re-adjust as soon as possible. It might even mean changing a goal because it no longer suits you. That is okay.

PLANNING AND EXECUTING YOUR FUTURE

The future will be there no matter what you do. You choose what that future will be for you. Where and what do you want to be in one year, two years, five years, ten, twenty? It is a great exercise to visualize that on a regular basis. There can be multiple futures for you. Tony Robbins[10] has a great exercise where you visualize your future if you don't do anything. You visualize the pain of continually feeling rejected and unloved because you did not solve the problem of finding love inside of you instead of looking for it outside of you. You visualize the pain of spending the next 20 years yo-yo dieting, seeing your body age prematurely, and looking old when you are still young. You feel the pain of losing your loved ones because you were miserable. You experience sadness because you did not do the rewarding career you always wanted. You are stuck in a dead-end job. And you grow old, sad, fat, and alone. This exercise is an awakening when done properly with all the pain and sadness of this alternate reality that could be yours. The great news is that it does not have to be your future. You can choose now what you want your future to be

---

[10] Tony Robbins: Personal Power

in one month, one year, five years, or more. Then you can redo this exercise as if you had conquered your relationship with food. How did it impact your life? Did the fact that you are happier, healthier and more energized have an impact on your relationship with your spouse or your children? Did you have the guts to go for a better career? Where are you in five, ten, or twenty years of living a healthy lifestyle? Where do you see yourself living? What kind of vacations do you have? This is a great exercise and its fun!. Do it regularly.

Everything you do today affects where you will be. I often used to excuse my behavior by saying, "It does not matter if I binge today. I will start again tomorrow." But it does matter. It matters a great deal because the problem is not the weight gain but the need for self-love and self-control, and a healthy body image. If you binge now, you are only confirming that you don't have self-love and you don't have a healthy body image. It's not congruent to your affirmations, dreams, and goals. You are lying to the one person in your life that is the most important person in your life: YOU. In order for you to change, you have to act, think, and live differently. That is the only way. And you know it works, you have been living, breathing, thinking self-loath and bad body image for years. It is not easy breaking a pattern of years, but the good news is that if your old way of living hurts bad enough, then you'll know you are ready to change it. So keep in mind that it is your choice. You are no longer a child. The time is now. Are you ready to commit 100%? Are you ready to choose your future?

Now, how do we go about it? The first thing to ask yourself is, "What do you want?" Do you have personal goals? Professional? Do you simply want great health? Make a list. You have to be precise in what you want and you have to put your wants into a timeline: "I want to be a size X by November 1st," or "I want to find my soul mate this year, and I want to marry him next year." At first, list everything that comes to mind—like a Christmas list. Then you can clean it up. Here are some examples:

HIGH LEVEL

Area of your life	Items	Date
Personal	Be two dress sizes smaller	November 1, 2012
Personal	Body Mass Index of 21	December 15, 2012
Personal	Be at peace with my relationship with food	Now
Personal	Find my soul mate ➢ Gorgeous ➢ Sense of humor ➢ Gentleman ➢ Intelligent	First quarter 2012
Material	Condo in San Diego	Second quarter 2013
Material	Fly first-class only	January 2013
Material	European cruise on the Queen Mary in a suite	Fall 2012
Career	Be a writer	Summer 2012
Career	Do a professional photo shoot for a major magazine	Summer 2012
Community	Do charity work: ➢ Serve dinners for the homeless ➢ Give 1% of my salary to charity	Now
Finance	Millionaire 5 million 10 million	By the time I am 50 By the time I am 55 By the time I am

Area of your life	Items	Date
		60

You get the idea. Put everything down, including the kind of relationship you want with friends, family, and colleagues.

The next step is to divide and conquer. When I start the year, I normally have a minimum of one goal per area of my life. Pick your top goals for the next 12 months and start breaking them down. Split the year into quarters (four quarters per year of three months each) and divide your top goals in those four quarters.

DETAILED PLAN

Goal	Plan	Date
Smaller dress size: November 1, 2012	1. Get a complete check up with my doctor. 2. Meet with a nutritionist. 3. Get a gym membership. 4. Work with one of the gym professionals to prepare an exercise plan that meets my goals. Meet with the nutritionist to re-evaluate.	Mid-July 2012 3rd week of July 3rd week of July End of July End of August
Be at peace with my relationship with food: Now	1. Act *as-if* now. 2. Find my beliefs and clean them one by one. 3. Find my patterns and clean them one by one. 4. Monitor and clean my	Now and ongoing

Goal	Plan	Date
	thoughts. 5. Visualize the future I want. 6. See a therapist if needed.	
Be a writer: **Summer** **2012**	1. Discover what type of writing I am interested in (fantasy, mystery, self-help books, health). 2. Set aside one to three hours a week to start drafting and writing. 3. Find people who have published, and ask how they did it. 4. Start researching publishing companies. 5. Can I write magazine articles to start?	Month 1 Month 2 Month 3 Month 4 Month 5

And so on and so on. During the course of the year, re-adjust. Maybe one goal takes precedence over another one. Maybe the actions you are taking are not helping you achieve your goal. Be flexible, be persistent, and stay focused. Do not beat yourself because you have to change a few things.

And act *as-if* you had it now.

Chapter 5 Summaries

> ➢ List what you expected after reaching your goal weight.
> ➢ Review and manage the list.
> ➢ Act *as-if* now.
> ➢ List your goals and put a date when they will be achieved.
> ➢ Divide and conquer—plan how to achieve your goals.

Chapter 6: It's Time to Do Some Clean Up

Wellness isn't about deprivation and it's not about perfection. It is about pointing yourself in the direction of growth, training yourself to get comfortable with your highest potential, and then taking small steps to support that shift. It's about showing up for yourself, day by day, and then one day finding that you've undergone a transformation.

KATHY FRESTON
New York Times best-selling author
who focuses on healthy living and conscious eating

Every time you grow, it changes something around you. The transformation you physically went through was not small. It was huge and it moved many things around. Some changes you noticed and some you did not. One obvious change is your relationship with others. You changed so obviously it changed. For example, you don't do happy hour at that Mexican restaurant anymore. You get up early to work out. You bring your lunch, or you agree to go to restaurants only where they have healthy choices. Want it or not, this affects the people around you.

So let's start with the people you live with. The people you choose to live with care about you, your health, and your well-being. It should be a given that they support you 100%, right? Wrong! You have disturbed the natural order of things established in the household. Just because you choose to eat healthy does not mean everyone has to! Here are a couple of scenarios to consider.

Scenario 1:

If it's only you and your spouse (or significant other), the first step is to speak to him in a nice relaxing setting. (I'll use "him" in this scenario because I went through this with my husband.). Don't have this discussion when you know he has had a bad day and he is stressed. Be sure to know beforehand what your aim is. Do you want to lose 20 pounds quickly for a specific event? (This is obviously not healthy.) Do you seriously want to be improving your lifestyle forever? (This is the healthy choice.) Your decision will affect him in different ways. He will want to know how it impacts his life, so it is important to involve him in the decision process. If you decide without his input that you are not doing the Friday night dinner anymore at the ribs place with those tasty fries or the movie with the jumbo popcorn, he will understandably be upset.

Discuss what your goal is, why you are doing it, and ask for his thoughts and opinions. If he says, "You're not fat," well, good for him. He has learned a few things over the years! If your goal is to improve your overall health then you already have an idea of what you want to do. Maybe you want to meet a nutritionist for a good start. Maybe you already did. Give him time to get up to speed with you. Chances are, you have been thinking about this for a while. He will either tell you that he is not interested in changing his habits, or that he is willing to change a couple of things, or perhaps that he is going in with you.

In any case, you need to find common ground and a plan that works for both of you. I was lucky; my husband supported me all the way. He has changed a couple of things, such as not bringing dessert into the house anymore or being careful not to make too many pasta dinners. He is the cook in the house, and I am lucky that he loves preparing meals with protein and vegetables and rice or rice noodles. I joined a gym that was a bit further away from home but that had a package deal with private training, a nutritionist, a spa, and a medical spa. My husband was understanding and accepted that I would be gone a bit more and that I would not be able to join him as often at our favorite bar. What you have to keep in mind is that you shouldn't try to change him. It is a big decision, and for it to work, it can only come from within. He might like the results on you and join in.

You know the quick gimmicks don't work. You can lose the 20 pounds for the high school reunion or the wedding, but it won't last because you did not do it for you. You did it for external gratification, and that never works.

What if he is not supportive? What if he keeps ordering the fried chicken and the fries and the double-layer chocolate cake that you love so much? Let him. But it will tell you something you may not want to know about him, especially if he tries to sabotage your efforts. You need to realize that if you change (and here is news: you are changing!), it will change the dynamic of you as a couple. He will accept the change or not. It is a chance you have to take for yourself. The good news is that, at this point, you have lost the weight and you now know where your spouse stands. Stick to your goals, but respect your spouse's choice.

Scenario 2:
You are a child in a family all living together. I am from a huge family so I understand the dynamic. I think the best thing to do is to have a family get together and discuss the options available for everyone involved in the process. If it is too much to do it all at once, meet them individually. Are they going to support and help you? Are they interested in getting on board? You will know quickly which way each individual is going to go. And focus on those who have a positive attitude towards your goals. If you feel they have a deeper interest, ask

for their opinions. If your parents are not health conscious, you may need to educate them or have a heart-to-heart with them. If the money is tight, there are ways to eat better without too much extra cost. You could go grocery shopping with your parent and find ways to eat better without spending more. You could even offer to pay for some extra stuff yourself and have a special section for you in the fridge and pantry. It will cost a bit more at McDonald's to order the salad instead of the $1 deal, but it is worth it. Offer to pay the difference there, too. If they are not supportive, find ways to get it done anyway without impacting their lives too much. You cannot choose your family, but you can learn how to deal with different personalities right there in your own home. It is a great test for life. You'll have to deal with different personalities everywhere; it is just a little more intense at home.

Now, let's look at reactions outside the home, whether it is at work, school, or in your social life.

I had to do quite a bit of clearing up of who I was hanging out with. As soon as you start seeing yourself in a better light, you realize that some people don't see you in that light. They don't see themselves or their lives in a good light and you are part of their environment. They will do everything to sabotage your new you because they aren't ready to change themselves. As far as I am concerned, now is a good time to clean up. They will use all kinds of tricks.

1. The guilt trip: "You don't have time for me anymore."
2. The sabotage: "You have lost enough weight. Have the French fries or the chocolate!" I hate that one! Don't they know that one bag of French fries can break the cycle of health I am embarking on? It is never the real healthy friends who offer you the bad food advice, either. Well, they can keep it!

3. The sympathy look: "You have worked so hard. Poor you. Have the cookies and the chips." A woman at my work kept telling me I looked tired. The thing was, I didn't. I had lost 25 pounds, I had tons of facials, my skin was tight and glowing, and I was getting all kinds of compliments from other people. I think she was just jealous and tried to put a downer on my success. These kinds of people are dangerous. They say things under the cover of love and friendship seemingly doing what is best for you, but they really aren't.

4. "You are so lucky!." I hate when people say that to me. The amount of work that I had to put into this success has nothing to do with luck. I will never again say to someone, "You are lucky.." It really has nothing to do with it.

Now let's look at the good folks that help you in your quest. My best friend and maid-of-honor at my wedding is a health fanatic. She is extremely conscious of her workouts and what she eats. I don't think I will ever go as far as she does. She does a detox that is a lot harder than I do, and she is a vegetarian. She is healthy and looks great. People turn around when she walks by (and now me too, yé!). She would never say to me, "Have the pasta and the dessert. You deserve it." She knows what it takes to look great. It is constant, never-ending healthy choices every day. Everyone needs to surround themselves with friends like this.

At work or at school, it can get nasty (especially at school) because you want to be part of a group and changing a group's dynamic may have some undesired effects (in retrospect, however, there are good effects). Again, it's a choice. If you are with a group whose goals or values are different than yours, change group. Easier said than done, I know. But it does not have to happen overnight. Take small steps. Get used to your new you. Start finding things you enjoy and find people who enjoy the same things. Instead of focusing on the negative (leaving an old group of friends), focus on the positive (finding new friends). If you want to be more active, find a team sport. Things will flow naturally. I joined the volleyball team in high school and college, and we even competed at the state levels. It saved my life because I had started to hang out with the wrong crowd and needed new friends. Your old gang might feel sad, angry, jealous, and resentful, but life goes on. They will have new friends and so will you. You may even have an old friend ask you for advice because she wants to do what you did and she is amazed at your results. Always keep the door open to help out others who see what you did and need guidance. Make sure people don't take advantage of you, but do help out. Wouldn't you have liked to have had someone helping you out? And if you did have someone to help, wasn't it good? It is an amazing feeling when you help someone become his or her best self.

I make it sound very easy to leave relationships that no longer suit you, but I know it is not. It took me months to act on the last relationship I was in that did not suit who I was anymore. You really have to follow your heart and act in your own time. In that case, I knew that I had outgrown the relationship, but there was a lot of time between realizing it and the actual act of leaving the relationship. I needed time to assimilate the new information. It does come as a shock. You may say, "Wow! Where did that come from?" Then you start thinking about it. You start seeing behavior (yours and person's) you did not see before. You start weighing the pros and cons of staying or leaving. Eventually things will settle one way or the other. You will stay if leaving frightens you. You will leave if you feel you have grown and the relationship just does not suit you anymore. It might be scary, but shouldn't you be more afraid of what would happen to you if you stayed?

I have to say two things at this point. One: Respect the time it takes you to get ready to reach the "I'm taking action timeline". You will know when you reach that point, and you will know if you are procrastinating. Don't procrastinate. It kills the momentum and the energy. There is a door, open it and jump through it! Second: Nothing bad ever came out of me leaving a relationship that I had outgrown. On the contrary, amazing things have happened. Letting go of someone or something that no longer fits the new you creates space for new things. I found I had space for better jobs and an amazing spouse. And I felt freer to live my life and take chances where before I would have analyzed things to death and not moved an inch.

Sometimes you want to stay because it is comfortable. However, if you are on the road of self-discovery and self-improvement, being comfortable is not what you want. Look at the people you hang out with or are living with and imagine yourself in one, five, and ten years. That should help you decide whether a change is needed or not. Sometimes, you may realize you've given control of your life to a person: they choose what is best for you. You may even think that you are the one making the decisions, but when you analyze it, you realize that you have been manipulated for years. Because these are huge decisions that will have a lot of impact on your life, it helps to write things down in your journal. It helps organize your thoughts and feelings and helps you make the right decision. And even if I said that you shouldn't procrastinate, you do not want to rush through things either. Writing in your journal will help you get a grip on what is going on. One last thought on this: Don't let others pressure you into doing something you are not ready for. Sometimes peer pressure is strong and it is difficult not to follow. But it's important; you have to follow your own heartbeat.

CLEANING UP OLD THINGS

Now that we have covered people, let's talk about things. It is cathartic to clean out your clothes. I had eight different sizes of clothing in my closet. When I told my therapist I wanted to clean them out, she asked if I was sure because I might gain the weight back! I was devastated to hear someone who understood the psyche so well say such a horrible thing to me. Granted, over the years she had seen my weight fluctuate over and over, but I was hurt that she did not believe as much as I did that this was the last time. Well, I decided to see it as a test for me to find out how resolved I was. And I was and I am. You never know where negative comments will come from. They might even come from someone who cares about you.

Let's go back to cleaning out your closet. I don't mean just get rid of the big clothes (an amazing feeling, by the way). I mean re-evaluate how you want to look today and tomorrow (the act *as-if* part). For example, if you want to become an executive, buy a suit and look like an executive. Part of acting *as-if*, however, is being comfortable with who you are. All my life, I have seen women who wear low-cut tops to work. Every once in a while, I wore one, and I just felt self-conscious. So I made a decision. I got rid of everything in my closet that made me uncomfortable. I did keep some low-cut tops, but I'd leave those for dates with my husband. Why insist on wearing something I was not comfortable with just because it is fashionable? The trick is to decide who you want to be and how you want to feel and then dress to make it happen. At the office, I want to feel confident, self-possessed, and respected. In order to feel that way, I dress in suits and button-up shirts. When I am out with my husband, I want to feel feminine and sexy. A co-worker once saw me at the end of the day on Friday when I was on my way to a date. He asked why I didn't dress like that at the office. I replied that at the office I was there to work. I didn't need to be distracted by the way I look or the reaction I was causing. That is my view. It is not right or wrong, but I know it is right for me. That is what you need to figure out for yourself.

Now, what else can you clean up? By the way, I certainly believe in charity, so make sure to give those things away to a good organization. I think the next step is your books and paperwork. It has nothing to do with having lost weight, but it has a lot to do with letting go of your old self.

The first place to look is through your old school books and notes. I have kept a book but not all the notes. I know I will never look at those again. My husband sometimes finds that I am too quick to throw things out. He is right because I have forgotten I've thrown something out and gone to look for it. Again, do what is right for you. Another thing to look at is memorabilia from old boyfriends or ex-husband. Do you throw it out? That is up to you. It can feel good to get rid of some stuff, such as old photo albums (although that might be less of a problem with digital photos). This cleaning up process is important. It empties some areas of your life and leaves space for better things to come.

YOUR CALLING

Do you feel you are in the wrong place? Are you fulfilled with what you do every day? In the spirit of being your best self and who you were meant to be, those are important questions. Never in my life have I asked myself those questions as much as I do now. A lot of time is spent working, so it is important to be happy working. Imagine all the energy wasted if you go to work unhappy day in and day out. Find your calling, your passion. Your work may be your calling, but it does not have to be. It can be your hobby and that is okay. If your work is fine and you are not unhappy with it, it pays the bills, and you have a hobby that thrills and drives you, then all is good. For other people, their work needs to be their calling. I believe I am in that category.

The big question to ask yourself is: What your calling is? This is not always easy to answer. Some people know right away and others, like me, don't. A couple of tricks to get to know what it is, is listing what you love to do, what makes you feel good and happy, and what makes you unhappy. Also, you may find that your calling when you were 20 years old may differ from your calling when you are 40 years old. What makes me happy now is different than what made me happy years ago. Spend time evaluating if you need to change things in your career. The same goes for your environment. Are you happy with where you live (your home and your neighborhood)? Do you feel you need to get away from your home or get away from winters? Think about everything that makes you unfulfilled or unhappy.

The conclusion to this chapter is simple (although not that simple to act upon): follow your instinct and ask the right questions. End it and clean it.

Chapter 6 Summaries

> ➢ Review your relationships. Are they good for you?
> ➢ Clean up those old drawers and closets.
> ➢ Dress the way you want to feel.
> ➢ What is your calling?
> ➢ Are you happy in your current environment?

Chapter 7: Enough with the Guilt and the Worry

There's always going to be bad stuff out there. But here's the amazing thing—
light trumps darkness, every time. You stick a candle into the dark,
but you can't stick the dark into the light.

JODI PICOULT
An American author who was awarded the New England
Bookseller Award for fiction in 2003

GUILT

Let's start with guilt. Guilt is such a heavy feeling, isn't it? It takes you down; it makes you feel like you are a bad person. There are many kinds of guilt. Sometimes it is guilt that you carry around for years, and sometimes it is today's guilt of saying "No." There are plenty of books out there about how to say "No," but let's focus first on the old guilt. I felt guilty about not treating my younger brother well when we were young. One summer he spent some time in a hospital, very sick, and I never went to see him. He mentioned it to me when we were adults, and I felt guilty about it. He said not to worry, but I know it hurt him and he buried that hurt deep inside. I do like my brother. He is one of my favorites in my family. He did not have it easy, being the last one of ten kids, and I am proud of him. He stands up for himself, and he has a nice family against all kinds of odds. For those reasons, I asked him to walk me down the aisle at my wedding. It was a proud moment for both of us. I see the pictures of that day, and he truly looks happy and proud to have done it. I believe that I have resolved the guilt issues I had with him, and I am happy about that. One important thing to know about guilt is that you can only control your side of things. If you did hurt someone you care about and you apologized and made it up to them then you can feel good about yourself. If they did not or will not get over it, that is their problem, not yours. There is nothing you can do about that. Walk away. They will only drain your energy.

One cause of my guilt was success. I would feel guilty if I succeeded. In order to avoid that feeling, I avoided being too successful. I was just successful enough to not feel guilty about it. It is like I had an unknown threshold. That was one more wrong belief that I worked on changing. Isn't it amazing the things you discover about yourself when you dig a little? A few years ago, I would have never thought that I felt guilty about being successful. I had a belief that because I was one of the youngest in my family that being successful belonged to the older ones, not me. The guilt also comes from growing up with very little money. If I became wonderfully successful, like a multi-millionaire, wouldn't people come and want a piece of me, like when you win the lottery? I focused on the problems of being rich instead of the advantages of being rich. It is amazing. It's like looking at all the negatives of winning the lottery. I needed to get back to my current really. I needed to focus on what was real. I am a good and generous person, and I would handle any lottery winnings fairly. I should not even worry about it. It goes back to my old desire to please everyone and hating to say no. What do you do about guilt?

There are some steps you can follow.

1. List to your guilty feelings and then look at one guilt at a time.
2. Review and analyze each one.
3. If it is an old guilt towards someone you care about, call them, write to them, explain where you are at, and resolve the issue with them. I will talk a bit more about this subject in the chapter about forgiveness.

4. If the person has passed away, write a letter anyway to clear the air for yourself. If the issue is too heavy for you, see a therapist.

5. If it is an old guilt towards someone you don't particularly like, you can follow Step 3 (because you are doing it for yourself not them) or write a letter and burn it.

6. For the daily guilt of not being able to say "No" when you want to, start small. Pick a small thing and say "No." Build up to bigger issues. Momentum is a wonderful tool to use here. I used to have problems with authority figures. I was never able to say "No" to my bosses when they wanted me to take on a project or do overtime. I started small. I also had to weigh the pros and cons of saying "No" to new projects. You have to accept the repercussions on your career.

Keep an eye on your feelings when doing this exercise. You know what feels right and what feels wrong. You don't want to start saying "No" to everyone. That would be the other extreme. Remember that we live in a society, and we have to deal with other people all the time. I believe that guilt is linked to a lack of self-esteem. Give yourself the place you deserve in your life. Stop giving all that space to work, friends, colleagues, husband, wife, kids and none for yourself. Like everything else, start small and build up. When that feeling of guilt creeps up on you, talk to it and joke with it. You could even create an affirmation to say for 30 days.

WORRY

Worry is a dream killer. You really need to work on resolving this issue in order to move on because the energy you spend worrying all the time is not time well spent. Use this time instead to confirm and work towards your goals and visualize. Let's take one step at a time. It took you years to build this worry attitude; it won't disappear right away. And, as in everything, you have to know where you are before looking at how to get to where you want to be. I used to worry all the time about everything. It is a label I had given myself: worrier.

I used to worry about
  ➢ gaining weight
  ➢ not having the perfect body
  ➢ not impressing my boss (or any father figure)
  ➢ not being loved by everyone
  ➢ About what people would think if I did this or that
  ➢ getting lost while driving
  ➢ missing my airplane connection
  ➢ having a bad seat on the plane
  ➢ not being liked by my employees
  ➢ not getting a good spot to sit at the pool or at the beach when I am on vacation

You name it, I worried about it.

I am better than I used to be. My husband is not a worrier, so I have learned a lot from him. Why worry about something that you have no control over? True, but let's separate the good worries from the bad ones.

  1. If you are worried about a job well done or delivering a good speech or doing great on an exam, those are good worries. A good worry forces you to see the areas you need to work on and prepare to succeed. For example, look at being worried about a tough exam. First of all, never bring yourself down with bad thoughts—"It's too tough," "I am not that smart," "I will fail." Control your thoughts, remember? If you are in that class, doing the exam, it's because you deserve to be there and you were meant to be there and you can succeed. Now, roll up your sleeves and start studying. Break it

down into mini-goals. Do the stuff that is harder for you first, but be sure to put some easy stuff in there so you don't go nuts. If it's too hard, get help. Do everything you can to get ready for this exam so that once you have written it, you can proudly say you have done everything in your power to get ready for it. What I am saying in this case is that worry (when managed properly) can be a driving force for success. This goes as well for work. If the work project is too big, break it down into smaller projects and attack one after the other. Think about delegating or asking a colleague for help. The worry about giving a speech is a common one. I have it as well. The best way to alleviate the stress and worry is to practice, practice, practice. You can start by practicing alone, but then practice in front of people to gather constructive criticism. There are classes you can take if you want to be great at it. But no matter how many classes you take, you still have to practice alone and in front of people to get better. John F. Kennedy was not a good speaker when he started going around Massachusetts to become a congressman. Luckily, he had his whole family to offer constructive criticism in order to improve, and, my God, he did.

2. The second kind of worry is when you feel your safety is at risk. Follow your intuition and be street smart. If you park in an underground parking garage and you have to pick up your car at one in the morning, keep your wits about you (and maybe find a better place to park your car). Worrying about walking at night in a bad neighborhood is a good kind of worry.

Like everything, your worry has to remain in check in order to serve your positively. If you worry so much about your safety that you never get out of the house, then that is another problem entirely for which you need professional help.

Let's get to the other kinds of worry.

I am always worried I will gain the weight back. I have always said that losing the weight is easy but maintaining it is hard. What can I do to remove this worry? The best thing to do is form healthy habits for life. I don't worry about brushing my teeth or removing my makeup at night. Those healthy habits are ingrained in my routine. I do those things automatically, and I don't worry about them at all. So what do we do first? Get rid of the old belief. It is just a belief and it is not serving you well.

Using my worry over weight gain as an example, let's break it down and see where I can take some positive actions and patterns I can reinforce. Let's look at a typical good day. I have blueberry or strawberries with flax seeds and crushed almonds and almond milk for breakfast. It has fruits, healthy fat, and protein. Sometimes I have a big fruit salad instead and have all my portions of fruit in one sitting to ease up the digestion by not mixing it with other food. I don't like eggs and am gluten intolerant, so I don't have regular bread or cereal. I found a healthy corn-based, non-gluten cereal that is good, and I have it every once in a while. I have yet to find good non gluten bread that is not frozen! Breakfast for me is never an issue. A healthy breakfast is a habit because I developed a good pattern. My mid-morning snack is fruits or vegetables with a protein. Lunch consists of leftover dinner or a salad or sushi or a simple soup meal (rice noodles, chicken or beef, and vegetables). For drinking during the day, I have either green tea or decaf coffee (with almond milk) and lots of water. I cut all the sodas from my diet. I may have one a month (diet, of course!). Now we get to the tricky part for me. By the time the afternoon arrives, I am more vulnerable. That is when I get the urge to eat cookies or a couple of chocolate bars. I am also vulnerable at night: I love to have a big dinner. Those are bad patterns. I needed to implement better patterns, such as eating more often. Instead of three big meals, I should eat something healthy every two or three hours. I could also have a bigger breakfast or bigger mid-morning snack so I don't get so hungry in the afternoon and at dinnertime.

I tend to eat most of the time with these new patterns. And now I prefer smaller meals every two or three hours. It is important to me to never have a stomach that is so full that I can barely breathe. You know the feeling; you go to your favorite restaurant and have the bread, the salad, the pasta dish, the dessert. You are so full you can barely walk out the door. I also find it secures me to have food at regular intervals. The small meals give me a sense of security and well-being.

The other action I have taken is regular exercise. I have to do it every day. It stabilizes me. I used to work out in the morning, but I like to write early in the morning so now I work out at night. I also try to go for a walk at lunch when it is nice outside, and I walk to work and back.

Keeping my weight at my goal weight is totally feasible, but it still requires focused attention. Sometimes I complain and cry out, "Why is this so hard?" I have to remember that it is my choice, and I have to deal with it. I could be 20 pounds heavier, and it would be easier to maintain, but that would not please me. I just have to stop complaining and move on. The trick is to make sure you find a healthy weight that makes you feel and look great. I am conscious of the fact that I am in my forties and I will never look like I'm in my twenties. My God, in my twenties, I didn't look like I was in my twenties! In order to stay in my bracket, I weigh myself once a week. And if I have gained a bit, I react right away to bring it back down. I think this is important because if you let it slide, it will be harder to get it back. Sometimes I get upset that it requires so much work, and I envy those people who seem to get things so easily. But I need to stop envying people, because when you dig a little, it wasn't so easy for them, either. They had to be persistent in their efforts and focus their energies on the task at hand. They also had to take a leap of faith. I am thinking of the likes of Jack Canfield, Oprah, Coco Chanel, and Tony Robbins. None were a success overnight, but they really believed in themselves and that helped.

So stop it right there, stop envying others who make things look easy. Become one of those people who makes it look easy. Accept that it takes consistent and focused effort to remain thin and toned. For me, accepting this removes the worry. I replaced the worry with strong self-knowledge. I can get it done, and there is no doubt in my mind that I can do it. I certainly know what to do to accomplish my goals. Looking at strong people, and reading their biographies helps me stay focused. Worrying involves self-doubt, but I have plenty of examples around me that tell me I can succeed when I follow the basic steps outlined here.

- Remove the worry by creating a new belief.
- You are not a worrier. You are a doer.
- Remove the worry by taking action and changing your patterns.
- Remove the worry by putting a plan in place and following it consistently.
- Remove the worry by putting yourself in a place where losing is not an option.
- Remove the worry by visualizing how amazing your life is right now without worry and how amazing it will be for the next five, ten, or twenty years.

I believe 100% that when you stop worrying about everything in your life and stop feeling guilty, your life will improve. You will feel less stressed and you will feel more in charge of your destiny; you won't feel like you are letting others decide how you should feel and who you are.

Chapter 7 Summaries

- ➢ What do you feel guilty about? Make a list.
- ➢ What do you worry about? Make a list.
- ➢ Solve each issue one step at a time.

Chapter 8: From the Inside Out

Growing into your future with health and grace and beauty doesn't have to take all your time. It rather requires a dedication to caring for yourself as if you were rare and precious, which you are, and regarding all life around you as equally so, which it is.

VICTORIA MORAN
An American writer and speaker, specializing
in books on spirituality and nutrition

How do you get started? By finding out where you are at! The first few chapters in this book gave you a glimpse of who you are and where you are at. Let's dig a little deeper.

WHERE ARE YOU AT

<u>Physically</u>
Have a complete physical test done. In addition to a regular medical physical (blood pressure, diabetes, etc.), be sure to test and calculate your bone mass, the percentage of fat and water in your body, your metabolic age, and your aerobic capacity. These numbers will give you something concrete to work with. Assuming you have no major medical problems, you can now work on goals besides your weight on a scale. You have starting points for all sorts of goals. Here are my results measured at my physical check up at the gym, by my personal trainer:

Category		Goal and comments
Body Fat	38%	A healthy body fat percentage for women is between 25% and 30%. A good goal target is 27%.
Body Water	45.7%	A healthy body water percentage is around 60%. Drink a lot of

Category		Goal and comments
		water each day: 2 liters.
Visceral Fat	7 lbs.	Visceral fat is the fat that surrounds your organs. A healthier amount would be four to five pounds.
Bone mass	5.4 lbs.	For a woman between 110 and 165 pounds, a bone mass of 5.3 pounds is average.
Metabolic age	60	This is a calculation of how well your body uses energy for your age group. I have a metabolic age almost fifteen year older than my chronological age!
Muscle mass	103 lbs.	A good amount of muscle is 108 to 110 pounds.
Cardiovascular training	Poor	I could not walk up a flight of stairs without breathing hard. A good goal is to be able to do thirty minutes of aerobic activity at around 80%. However, a simple way to start is by simply walking and taking the stairs wherever possible. Pedometers are widely available to help you track your steps (and give you extra motivation). Aim for 10,000 steps a day. The Fit Bit app is also a great tool. Take it slow—you'll enjoy it more and stick with it longer. Do only as much as you feel comfortable with each day. And be sure to consult your doctor before starting any exercise program.
Flexibility	average	Some people are naturally more flexible than others. But, stretching and working on flexibility is something that should be incorporated into your

Category		Goal and comments
		routine. Again, stretching should feel good. Don't push it. Let your body ease into it.
Specific health problems	knees and back	Be kind to your weak points. I could not do high-impact aerobics because of a lack of cartilage in my knees. I must also be careful of an old back injury and take time to stretch and strengthen that area whenever possible. Chiropractors, osteopaths, and physiotherapists can help you work around specific physical limitations or health issues (e.g., diabetes).

So in summary, I need less fat, more muscle, a better metabolic age, and more cardiovascular training. To combat my lack of body water, I needs to look at nutrition (including allergies, intolerances, and other medical issues).

A good way to discover your own allergies or intolerances is to do a detox. As allergies are usually quite obvious, you may already know which allergies you have. Intolerances are harder to detect. I did a supervised ten-day detox before slowly re-introducing foods I had suspicions about. I thought I had issues with dairy. I didn't think I was allergic to it, but dairy created so much mucus in my respiratory system that I always felt like I had a cold or sinusitis. I'll talk a little more about detox in the chapter about treatments.

I also had my suspicions about gluten because a lot of members of my family have celiac disease (extreme reaction to gluten). I have an intolerance. It is not extreme, but there are times where my body rejects it. In general, gluten makes me balloon up. I don't digest it very well. Oddly enough, while

I was trying different grains in order to avoid gluten, I discovered I have a much stronger intolerance to quinoa!

So there you are. Knowing what you have to work with physically is helpful. And if your last medical physical was years ago, you need to have another. You need to know where you are right now before you can know where you are going.

Mentally

The past few chapters have concentrated on preparing yourself mentally for losing the weight and keeping the weight off, but let's look at your mental state in terms of getting started. Multilayer, remember?

When I embarked on my weight loss for the wedding, I did what is called a "boot camp." They are nice to kick off any new program to improve your health, but for someone like me who wanted to lose the weight for external validation, they are dangerous. It gave great results, but deep down I knew that in my head, unconsciously, there was no way I could keep up "boot camps" forever. I had a plan to follow up after the wedding, but I was tired—I had worked so hard—and had already felt the satisfaction of obtaining my goal weight for the wedding. The result was that I started slipping here and there and, in the end, gave up and regained the weight.

So before you start, here are some important questions you have to ask yourself to find out where you are mentally:
  ➢ Why are you losing weight?
     ○ For yourself?
     ○ For others?
     ○ For an event?
     ○ To be healthy and/or thin for a short period of time?
     ○ To be healthy, strong, flexible, and your best self forever?

- o Because you are tired not being your best?
- o Because you know you are not who you are meant to be?
- o Other reasons?
- ➢ What are your bad patterns?
  - o Emotional eating is an example of a bad pattern
- ➢ What beliefs do you have that limit you?
- ➢ What areas of your life are you unhappy with?
  - o Career?
  - o Love?
  - o Family and friends?
  - o Community?
  - o Home?
- ➢ What are you willing to do for the rest of your life?
- ➢ Why have you not taken responsibility for your life so far?
  - o Who have you been blaming?
  - o What past event have you been blaming and/or focusing on?
  - o In your everyday life, are you the victim or the hero? Why?
- ➢ Why is it more painful to lose the weight and be healthy than not lose it?
- ➢ What is currently going on in your life that is stressful (good or bad)?
  - o Is there an event that is coming up that is stressful?
  - o Are there big things happening at work or within your family?
  - o Are you going to see someone who upsets you?
- ➢ Are your thoughts helping you or sabotaging you?
- ➢ What have you done in the past that has worked?
  - o Changing a habit and/or pattern?
  - o Changing a belief?
  - o Losing weight?
  - o Feeling great one day?

> ➢ Make a list of all your successes since you were a child. This will help to show you that you have done great things in your life.

Wow, the above list is a mini–therapy, in itself isn't it? Your body and mind are wonderful. If you are overeating, binging, drinking to excess, doing drugs, overworking, stressing out about performing, or hurting yourself in any way, shape, or form, it is because you are not happy in some area of your life. You are not satisfied. You are not who you feel you are meant to be. Something or someone is in your life that does not belong. Something or someone should be in your life that you are missing. You get the idea.

Start slowly. Go through the questions in your journal and start making lists. Review and analyze everything. Your journal is your best tool, but for this chapter, you may find it easier to use a computer where you can make tables and compare things. You don't have to do everything on the same day—you did not get to where you are in a week. It may be difficult not to be impatient. If you're excited about changing, you would like it to happen right now. There have never been truer words spoken than "the journey is as important, if not more, than the end result."

This task may seem huge but you cannot get around it. If you want to solve it from the inside out, you need to know what is inside. At any given time, if you feel what you discover is too painful, seek the help of a therapist; they know what they are doing.

After regaining the weight, I realized I wanted to lose the weight from the inside out. I wanted to understand and resolve the reasons behind my emotional eating. Basically, if it was not for my binging during emotional episodes, I would be just fine. I like to work out—even if sometimes I need to kick myself in the butt to get out there—and I like healthy food. I knew where to put my focus. I went through all the questions in detail, and I found all kinds of answers, very helpful answers. As soon as you slip, you need to go back and ask yourself specific questions to find out why.

At the base, I had a self esteem problem. I had to work on strengthening it. It is not a big surprise that mind and body are intimately and permanently linked. You have to work on both together. This is why this list of questions is important. It will help you find out what is going on behind the scenes— find out what you are not paying attention to. Fast diets and fitness boot camps do not work if you don't fix what is in your head as well.

Find the triggers or patterns that are preventing you from achieving your goal and the reason you continually fall off the wagon. You take one issue at a time and resolve it as shown in earlier chapters. Some will be easy and some will be harder because you may not be ready. But the one thing to keep in mind is that failing is not an option. As soon as you leave one door ajar, it is like an option to fail, and your old self will find a way to open that door wide open and run in there. So close it shut. You really need to approach this with an attitude of determination and self-love. You cannot beat yourself up when you discover you need the junk food, for whatever reason. You need to fill yourself with love, understanding, and forgiveness. Realize that you created this self-preservation mechanism in your past, and it may have helped you, but it no longer serves you. It is actually armful now. Be thankful that you were smart enough back then to find this mechanism. But now, replace it with a healthy pattern. Feel thankful each step of the way. The self-loathing you may have had for yourself needs to be replaced with self-love and understanding. You need to change your attitude now, not when you are thin.

These questions will make you more aware of yourself. The hardest thing sometimes is to realize that you have fallen into a bad pattern. Patterns may happen so slowly and feel so natural that you may find yourself saying, "Oh God! How did that happen?" You have to remain focused. I am not kidding. By the end of this exercise, you should be well on your way to know the answers to the following questions:

> ➢ Why do you want to lose weight?
> ➢ Why are you behaving this way?
> ➢ What are your bad patterns and limiting beliefs?
> ➢ What are you willing to do to get to where you want to go?
> ➢ Do you want to keep on being a victim or be your own hero?

Now that you know where you are, let's review where you want to go and take the following as an example on how to proceed.

WHERE ARE YOU GOING AND HOW ARE YOU GOING TO GET THERE?

Let's clarify where to go, and, specifically, how to get there.

1. I don't want to lose weight. I want to have a healthy relationship with food. I want my choices to elevate me, not bring me down. I want to feel pride, happiness, strength, and courage every day. I want to feel healthy; I want to be healthy. I want to feel strong and be ready to take on the world every day. I want this in my mind and in my body. I want this for the rest of my life.
2. I have a list of my patterns and beliefs that need to be changed to match who I am and who I want to be. I update this list as I keep improving.
3. I monitor my thoughts, and I keep improving them to match who I am and who I want to be.

4. I am willing to face my fears. Changing my pattern of going for food when feeling anxious scares me. It has been a crutch since I was very young. How am I going to live without it? But I am willing to face changes that are required in my life in order to achieve my goal. If it means changing the people around me that are not good for me or if it means changing my job that I have had for fifteen years and my big, corporate title for something I find rewarding and fulfilling every day, I am willing to do it.

5. I am willing to make the effort to learn about and improve my nutrition. I am willing to understand that for my overall well-being, I need to work out every day. Exercise gives me a sense that I love myself, and it helps me to get in touch with my body.

6. I am willing to be focused and flexible. If something does not work, I am willing to analyze it and change it.

7. I am willing to involve specialists to help me achieve my goals. Why not use the knowledge and experience of people trained in their fields to increase my chances of success?

8. In order to have a clear idea of what I want, I have written down my goals on paper and list a date by which I want to reach them. I want to go by what feels right for me.

Goal	Elements	Date
Change the pattern of: No more emotional eating	Follow the instructions in Chapter 2. Create a healthy pattern: go for a walk, breathe, have a cup of herb tea, call a friend, write in my journal, etc.	Now
Check in	Every morning: Review my resolve and be grateful for what I have in my life.	Now

Goal	Elements	Date
Reflect	Every day: Monitor my thoughts and say my affirmations. List the thoughts that were not helpful. Analyze them and clean them.	Now
Take time to be happy	Put aside time every day for a little action that will make me happier. Find a career that is fulfilling and rewarding: update my CV, make some calls, list my interests, etc. Treat myself: take a bath, get a pedicure, and have a facial. For each area of my life that needs improvement, I will create a list.	Now
Get physical	Bring body fat down to within average. Bring body water to a healthy level. Bring down visceral fat level by a few pounds. Improve cardiovascular endurance (able to do one hour of exercise at 80% heart rate capacity). Improve flexibility (overall and on specific trouble areas). Match metabolic age to chronological age. Increase muscle mass as needed. Take measurements now and retake them every month.	6 months (less or more if you are concentrating on other goals)
Nutrition	Remove intolerances (foods that make you feel unwell). Remove junk food from the house. (Some may be able to have it around, but many may find a complete ban more effective). Eliminate sodas (diet or otherwise). They are just too bad for me.	Now
Nutrition	Eat smaller portions, but eat more often. Eat fruits alone first thing in the	Now

Goal	Elements	Date
	morning. Eat vegetables at each meal (except breakfast). Eat lean meat. Have fish or seafood at least once a week. Find new and interesting ways to eat protein that does not involve meat or fish. Stop eating three hours before bedtime. Drink alcohol at celebrations only. Reduce caffeine. Discover ways to make healthy desserts that I'll enjoy.	
Exercise	Do something every day. Do different forms of exercise so you don't get bored. Walk everywhere (10,000 steps daily). Consider yoga and/or Pilates to increase flexibility and strength. Consider spinning classes (indoor bicycling in groups). Consider a home elliptical machine and home weights. Consider swimming at your local pool. Get a massage once a month. Enjoy sauna and steam baths. Meditate every day.	Now
Commit	Most people say, "Go easy on yourself," but that does not work. Massive change demands effort. Total commitment towards this plan is mandatory. Leave no option to fail. Feel free to change and improve the plan, of course, but stay 100% committed. Don't try to control everything. Eating or doing something that was not on	Now

Goal	Elements	Date
	track is a setback not a failure. Let it go. Move on, and get back on track. Don't feel guilty. Find ways to laugh at old patterns and laugh at life. ENJOY THE JOURNEY! Forget the end results—they will come on their own. Create positive affirmations that you can say to yourself multiple times a day.	
Stop and listen	Listen to my body. Time spent filling up with junk food is time spent not listening. Re-establish the communication. Listen to my mind. If thoughts keep coming back again and again listen to them, write them down, and analyze them. Fix them. Thoughts will keep coming back again and again until they are listened to and acted upon. Action is necessary to move to the next step.	Now
Know your weaknesses	Am I weaker when I am extremely tired? When I am sick? Does junk food become comfort food or food I think I deserve, being tired and weak? If I miss a meal or get too hungry, do I overeat when food arrives? Do I get moody, angry, and bossy? Do I eat anything I can find if I wait too long between meals? Should I carry around snacks to avoid overeating during the day? I need to keep my eyes open and see what other weakness I have.	Now
Log progress	I will continue to write in my diary. On weekends, I will do a complete analysis of the week. I'll see where I could have improved, where I did very well, and what, if anything, I should change in the	Now

Goal	Elements	Date
	upcoming week. At regular intervals, I will redo the physical tests and measurements, and I will review the analysis of my patterns, thoughts, and beliefs. I'll look at how I did, and I'll change anything that needs improvements.	

At this point, you should have a clear understanding of what you want. Why don't you write it in a contract format and sign it? On the Oprah Show, Bob Green suggested this. It is a great idea. Keep it around—in your pocket or purse—read it a lot and review it a lot. Don't hesitate to amend it and re-sign it if something is not working.

Your goal is to make these goals your top priority in your life. Why? Because right now, not doing it makes your life an unhappy one. Not doing it keeps you in the role of victim, and dependent on others for your happiness. If you are blaming others, you won't attain the level of self-respect and self-esteem that you want to reach. Visualize yourself attaining your goals. Think of how amazing you will feel a few months from now and for the years to come.

Chapter 8 Summaries

- ➤ Where are you at? Answer truthfully.
  - o Physically
  - o Mentally
- ➤ Where are you going?
  - o List everything that you want for yourself.
- ➤ How are you going to get there?
  - o It's time to make the detailed plan.
  - o Sign your contract to yourself.
- ➤ Get going. Be 100% committed.

Chapter 9: How to Not Gain Weight on Vacation: My Experience

To love yourself as you are is a miracle, and to seek yourself is to have found yourself, for now. And now is all we have, and love is who we are.

ANNE LAMOTT
A novelist and non-fiction writer

Well, let's go back in time a little bit. I had lost my twenty-five lbs, and I had an amazing wedding. I looked amazing in the dress. Now my new husband and I set off for our honeymoon in Maui. I was thinking how I was going to not gain weight on the trip. I had asked around, and everyone said it was not possible: "You cannot not gain weight on vacation." Well, I didn't accept that answer. I did eat more at the wedding—cake and all, but four days after the honeymoon, I was the same weight than I was on the day of the wedding. Contrary to what people say, it is possible to not gain weight on vacation and here is how.

The first obstacle was traveling day. You are not allowed to bring any food across borders, so I had to try to get decent food in the airport terminals. There are healthier foods in airports than in the past, but not many. I grabbed water and nuts. In the lounge—yes, bless my husband, we traveled mostly first-class—I found fresh fruits, low-fat yogurt, and granola. That was my first mistake. I am intolerant to dairy, but in choosing between intolerance and higher fat food, I chose intolerance. My body didn't forgive me. Within a couple of days, I started coughing like I had been smoking for thirty years and I develop a throat ache. After a few more days of dairy, I felt like I was choking. I felt like I had a sinus infection and my body started to feel bad overall. My choice to not gain weight overshadowed my body's own signals. It was a good example of me not listening to my body's needs. It was also a perfect example of what I wanted to change about myself with my new plan and my contract: I wanted to start listening to my body's needs. That was more important than a low-fat yogurt. I shouldn't force my body to digest something that it can't, just because I did not want to gain weight.

Back to the plane ride. For the first leg of the trip, we were in economy for a five and a half hour trip. I had brought along a bag of healthy nuts and a banana. I dozed off but in a bad position, and by the time we landed in Los Angeles, I had a neckache and the beginning of a migraine. My husband and I were also exhausted. On the night of the wedding, we went to sleep at five in the morning. I woke up at nine, unable to go back to sleep. We then had to get up at five in the morning to catch the plane, so I'd slept only nine hours in two nights. In Los Angeles, we had a three-hour layover before our next plane. I was miserable: hungry, tired, neck ache and migraine. We had soup and salad, but I felt so miserable at that point that all I wanted was comfort food. Being tired and sick is a weak point for me: I start to crumble. We made our way to the lounge where I found some Advil and my husband massaged my neck. He knows where my pain is, so he is good at alleviating it, but comfort wasn't instant. So I turned to my instant comfort: food. They had all kinds of food in the lounge, including cookies and those raisins covered with yogurt (yes, another good move on my part!). I temporarily turned into a cookie monster. I am not proud of that moment. The wait was so annoying. I just wanted to get there, already!

Finally, we got onto the next plane for another five and a half hour trip. But for this leg of the journey, we were flying first-class. The flight attendants were great. I don't know if it was because we are going to Maui, but everyone was nice, smiling, and relaxed. I felt better, but I was on a slippery slope at this point. I had a nice meal of shrimp, rice, and vegetables and white wine. I also gladly accepted the bread and the warm chocolate cookies. What is the point of being in first-class if you are not going to have those cookies? At this point, my adult self was wondering what happened. I was an alien to myself. Who was this girl? Where was the girl who left home that morning with all the right moves and beliefs? Well, I was exhausted. I think the wedding, the mad rush to lose the weight over the previous eight months, and the stress of not taking a decent vacation from work for almost a year, not to mention the eighteen hours of traveling got to me. It felt like all my good resolutions went out the window. Luckily, two glasses of wine and the great seats eased up my stress and my headache was almost gone by the time we landed in Maui. What could I do but put down an action for myself to work on getting through those hard moments without letting my younger self take over.

I would like to add a side note here. I had a choice to be pissed and upset at my mishaps or let them go, move on, regain my resolve, and enjoy our arrival in Maui. I could either embark on a guilt trip and a worry trip or let everything go and move on. I was good at feeling guilty about my setbacks. I was good at setting huge expectations for myself and when I didn't follow through, I was harsh with myself. But you cannot control everything. When things don't go exactly the way you plan, let them go. I learned to let them go and then, when I was in a quiet setting where I could think and write, I'd have a chance to re-evaluate the situation and get back on track.

So we get to Maui and our driver was waiting for us. Nice, chatty fellow. Thank God for my husband, who is a pillar of strength, because at that point I could not put two words together. We finally arrived at our hotel, and were welcomed with Hawaiian leis and cool drinks. They were quick and professional—not their first day. They knew their stuff, and we were quickly brought to our room with our luggage right behind us.

We had seen pictures of the room, but they did not do it justice. It was huge and amazing. It had a big terrace and huge bathroom. We loved it. It was only six in the evening, it was midnight to us. We were tired but didn't want to just go to bed, so we changed into summer clothes and went to the main lobby bar that overlooked the pool area and the beach. We had a drink and some light food. But by eight o'clock, we were in bed completely exhausted but tremendously happy.

We slept amazingly well, ten hours. Woke up refreshed and ready to visit the hotel and the area. Right then and there, I decided to forgive myself for the day before and move on. I did not want to enter into a negative spin. The place was amazingly beautiful and relaxing. We were there (finally) and I could relax, enjoy life, breathe, and take care of my body and my soul. The hotel had a great gym and a great spa. I found a scale in the spa so I hopped on. I promised myself not to be over that number before I left for home. We enjoyed our visit to the spa and had a great breakfast. I registered for a couple of spinning classes, and I hired a private trainer for a couple of sessions to make sure I stayed focused on my training. I didn't mind eating more as long as I could stay active and burn off those extra calories. The good thing was that I could do other activities, such as kayaking and swimming.

I knew that I needed to plan things out. It is a must. So I set out to advance this book, read from the series of *The Wheel of Time* (13 books in the series; each book is 900 pages), exercise, work on my tan a bit (although I am not crazy about lying in the sun for hours). We also wanted to see Pearl Harbor and the whales. But for the first couple of days we took it easy; we relaxed and slept almost ten hours a night for the first week. I wanted to relax and enjoy myself, but I also wanted to remain conscious of my choices and focused on my goal to not gain weight on vacation. I tried to find the balance between not being too strict, but also not having junk food (because having junk food is a flag that there are deeper problems).

A typical relaxing day when we didn't visit anything would follow a similar plan. I'd get up early (around six in the morning), make coffee in the room, and write for a couple of hours while eating fruits and almonds (I'd stopped eating yogurt!). I would go to the gym for an hour or so with or without a trainer, and then meet up with my husband. We would go over to the pool and find a cabana because I don't like to stay in the full sun. I'd read or write some more, and order a salad or a protein shake for lunch. Around mid-afternoon, my husband would go to the gym and I would continue reading and writing until it was time to get ready for dinner around seven in the evening. After dinner, my husband and I would go for a walk on the beach. That would be a typical day. I allowed myself alcohol in the evenings, although I stayed off booze altogether for a couple of the evenings. All in all, there was no secret to my success. I simply planned my day.

One day, we went to visit Pearl Harbor. That day started at six in the morning and ended at nine in the evening. Wow! Full day. I did not have a gym work out that day, but I did a lot of walking, I am pretty sure I walked over 10,000 steps. One problem I encountered was that we were not allowed bags or purses of any kind on the military base, and I need to eat several small meals every day. After our short flight to Honolulu, we took a tour bus to Pearl Harbor for the visit. It was an amazing place to visit; it brought me back to the basics, to what's important in life. But, the tour put me in a situation where I was hungry and had no food. I quickly became moody and bossy (you know like those characters on the "Snickers" commercials), and my husband vowed to always carry around a granola bar for me just in case!

After the visit to Pearl Harbor, we got back on the bus and visited some other places. We finally ended up at a restaurant we like, the Cheesecake Factory. After a lot of food, I was calm and collected again, but, unfortunately, I devoured bread and butter and way more food than I needed because I had waited too long before eating. I learned that I shouldn't go more than two or three hours without food. Even on vacation, I still prefer to eat more often but smaller meals. A mini-meal can be a vegetable and a protein or even just an apple. Not a full meal, just something to keep me going. Sometimes, just knowing I have food available is enough to calm me down.

It was a long day, and when I get tired and there is no place to relax alone, I tend to eat more. Looking on the positive side, I found and confirmed my areas of weaknesses, so I could plan in the future to counteract them.

I tried something while I was in Maui—a private meditation session. My only regret was that I tried it on my last full day there. Because anxiety makes me eat, finding ways to release stress and anxiety is important. I use exercise but I found that meditation also works. My teacher said that the best time to meditate is after a good jog—a good sweating session. Once I came back home, I kept up with the meditation every day. I find it does work better after exercise. The combination of the two has gotten rid some of my worst anxiety.

In summary, you can avoid gaining weight on vacation by following a few simple tips. Plan your day and be extra active because you will eat more on vacation. Try to avoid junk food and fatty desserts, and stick to wine rather than those fruity or creamy alcohol drinks. Take advantage of new and fun activities to do. Keep an eye on your weak spots. Also, try to stick with the good patterns you started at home, such as writing in your journal as often as you can. I found it helped to weigh myself at the resort at the beginning of the trip and to check in every four or five days. I am not a big fan of the scale, but it seemed to help me keep an eye on things. And, above all, don't forget to relax and enjoy yourself. Let go of the worry and the guilt.

Chapter 9 Summaries

- ➤ Plan ahead. Those long days of traveling are brutal.
- ➤ Keep active. Go to the gym, the pool, or the beach. Find new activities to do.
- ➤ Stay away from fruity and creamy alcohol drinks.
- ➤ Stay away from junk food and fatty desserts.
- ➤ Enjoy!

Chapter 10: Meditation and Visualization

The universe is always speaking to us....Sending us little messages,
causing
coincidences and serendipities, reminding us to stop, to look around,
to believe in something else, something more.

NANCY THAYER
An author of novels

I used to listen to Oprah and others talking about their *aha!* moments and wondered why I don't get those. You hear of people who encounter a moment that changed their life. Why not me? Well, I now know why. First of all, I did have those *aha!* moments. I just wasn't ready to see them. Second, I am a person who gets multiple *aha!* moments that culminate in a "Wow!" "Oh, my God!" or "How did I not see that?" moment. I don't think I ever had a huge *aha!* moment that changed my life, I think I had multiple moments. In retrospect, I see they could only have reached the pinnacle that they have.

For as long as I can remember, I was always split in two. I was in a place but felt out of place or I was focusing on my logical side but sad that I was ignoring my creative side. I was being moody and bitchy when I was basically calm and smiley. The day I left home, I decided that I had to rely on my logical side to survive and succeed. I pushed through my bachelor's and master's degrees even if I did not enjoy them. I pushed to have higher job titles because it seemed like it was my path. My therapist, who saw so much potential in me, pushed in the same way—for higher education and higher jobs. However, it became evident that there was a lack of balance in my life. I was so focused on logic and the left side of my brain that I forgot to relax and use my creativity and the right side of my brain.

When I became a vice-president, I was happy. I had finally made it, I was in an elite group, and I was sitting in on important meetings. I loved that about it. I can handle pressure, I can handle stress, I can manage projects and people, and I am good at it. But after a while, the honeymoon was over. I realized that at that level, I would only deal with problems: problems from the top and problems from the bottom. And I thought, "Wow. Is that it?" It was not so interesting anymore. I started thinking that I had done it all for nothing. It was also in a field that I was not passionate about, IT. I was there, I had made it, but I didn't like it. I didn't feel that it was my life's purpose. Well, all the studying and the hard, persistent work was not for nothing. I grew into who I am today because of it. How else would I have known that it was not for me if I hadn't done it! Besides, even if I was stuck in the wrong place, I could learn tons of things about myself.

Unfortunately, before I realized I was in the wrong job, I spent months getting angrier and angrier, and listening to myself less and less. We had the wedding and the honeymoon coming up, so I put aside all those feelings about work. I had to pay for the wedding right? Then we went to Hawaii. It was by far the most beneficial trip I had ever been on for two reasons: 1) I learned how to treat people, and 2) I learned about meditation.

Everyone who meets my husband speaks very highly of him. Why? He treats everyone with the utmost respect. And he does that even if he is tired, sick, angry, or fed up. No matter what, he treats people the way he likes to be treated. And people like to be treated with respect. For example, after a fourteen-hour day visiting Pearl Harbor and flying, our taxi driver felt like talking but I did not. I'm sure my husband was as tired as I, but he picked up the conversation with the driver. The driver was a nice man and loved Hawaii and loved to tell us all about it. I am sure that by the end of the ride, the driver must have thought that my husband was a nice man. My thoughts were simply that I was exhausted and I just wanted to relax in the back seat with my husband without that guy invading our space. After a day of recuperating, my husband and I talked about it. I had heard all the reasons for making an effort to be interactive and pleasant—you want to be treated the way you treat others or what you put out there comes back one hundred fold—but my husband simply said, "It is the only way to treat people." You treat them well, with respect and you care about their lives and their treating you will reflect the same. But that is not even why he does it. He does what he does because he is a respectable human being of the highest quality, and no matter how he feels, he cannot act any other way. And the way he acts reinforces who he is: a high-class human being. That got me thinking. Every time I treat someone with less than full respect, it means I accept two things: 1) I accept that others can treat me with less than full respect, and 2) I accept that I can treat myself with less than full respect. Even when someone is a jerk, my husband doesn't stoop to their level. He remains at his high-class level. Don't get me wrong, if someone is downright disrespectful to him or someone he loves, he will put them in their place, but respectfully. I am in awe of his self-control. I most definitely have to learn from him. So what I did after our talk was practice this new approach.

I was still in Maui, it was early in the morning, and I was on my way to the spa. On my way, I ran into a bellman in the elevator and started a conversation. He opened up right away, and seemed happy about our chat. At the spa, I discovered that they had made a mistake with my appointment. I got a bit bitchy with the lady and poof! she immediately became defensive and stopped smiling. This was amazing to me. In a span of less than ten minutes, I had tested my husband's theory, and he was, of course, right. It was amazing. Perhaps I knew all that but was not ready to see it. It was much easier to force my moods on others. But being harsh on others just brought my own mood down, not just theirs. I am actively working on this. It is not automatic, but the more I do it, the more it becomes natural. I can categorize this as an *aha!* moment.

The second thing I did, and oddly enough it was on the same day, was a private hour of meditating. The instructor spent a lot of time explaining things to me, and it was the first time anyone did. I always thought that meditating meant quieting your mind. The first thing he said to me was why on earth would someone ask the mind to perform something it was not meant to do. Right there he relaxed me because just the thought of trying to quiet my mind stresses me. He actually said that whatever came to my mind was okay. I should allow it and then release it. We went to a nice, quiet, secluded spot by the beach. He explained a few things and suggested two types of meditation: humming and ocean wave meditation. The type of meditation I learned and used on that day is irrelevant because everyone connects with a different form of meditation. If you want to learn more about meditating there are plenty of books and DVDs and schools to help you. What is relevant is that meditation, in whatever form you choose, should help you find a way to connect with your core self, your real self, the one without ego. God knows, I have tried over the years to meditate and quiet myself. I've tried to "hear" myself, but it never worked (I'll admit that I never did it consistently). I don't know why it worked in Maui. Maybe I was ready for it. Maybe it was the setting. Maybe it was the teacher. I was in paradise, and I had been there for two weeks, sleeping ten hours every night. I had no stress. The trick to meditation, however, is to be able to enter that calmness when everything is falling down around you. I am an overachiever, and I approached meditating with a desire to be the best. When the instructor told me that there is no right or wrong way to meditate, to just let it flow and feel it, it was relaxing for me.

First, we sat down. This was different from what I always thought about meditating. I thought it was while lying down. So sitting was an interesting change. The first fifteen minutes of the practice was a humming meditation. He said I needed to breath from the belly and to breathe in and breathe out while humming through my lips. I always used to laugh at this type of meditation, but not anymore. The vibration, through my lips and the rest of my body was amazing. I was actually disappointed when the fifteen minutes were up. There was music in the background and right after the humming was finished, we went into the ocean wave meditation. We breathed through the nose into the belly and breathed out through the mouth. When I breathed, I imagined a fresh ocean wave all over me, and when I breathed out, I imagined a warm wave removing all the toxins and stress and anxiety from my body. We did that for fifteen minutes as well. Once we'd done both meditations, he suggested another five or ten minutes to let me retake my body. By the way, we visualized an empty vase while meditating. With my eyes closed, I imagined looking on the inside of an empty vase. It was empty in the sense that I was letting go of all pain and stress.

The instructor said something interesting while explaining the process to me. He said that when you are stuck on a given feeling in your heart (pain, sorrow, sadness, or anger) and you keep it there, it prevents the flow of your heart as well as the next feeling that is waiting to come. I like the visual of an empty vase because it helps you to create space to let new things enter your life. That is what meditating does for me. It helps me go through emotions that are stuck. Imagine the happiness and joy that is not coming into your life because you are stuck on old pain and anger.

On the last morning in Maui, I had a craving for a huge carb breakfast. I decided to meditate for fifteen minutes using the ocean wave meditation technique. I was so calm after that, that I ordered a powder protein shake and fruits instead. I found it works. I meditate and focus on the empty vase and it opens up the day for me. By the way, did you know that "Zen" means being here and now?

After my meditation session, the instructor and I spoke and he told me about how important it is every day to find some private time to be quiet with your core self. It helps to find answers. It also helps when you feel you are not where you are supposed to be. I thought it was odd when he said that because I'd realized that I was not happy in the corporate world. During our talk, he told me that his sister had mentioned that she found that the first six months of her pregnancy were hard work but the last three months were all about letting go and letting things happen. In those last months, there is nothing else to do but take good care of yourself. Life will do the rest. To me, it meant that I can do all the groundwork and get ready for the life I want, but eventually I need to surrender. Surrender to life; it knows what to do next.

I felt that I had wasted too many years not listening to myself. There is so much noise out there—technology, radio, phone, TV—you feel pulled outside of yourself. You need to focus on being grounded, centered, and need to develop a strong core. If you do this, life will come to you instead of you running to be everywhere at once. It is exhausting to try to be everywhere, to learn all the new technologies that come up every day, and to meet the right people who will help you get ahead. You keep searching for answers out there when, in fact, the only place to find them is within you. You just have to be quiet enough to hear them.

I listened to Oprah's magnificent last show and she said just that—stay still. Anytime she has to make an important decision, she stayed still and asked herself for the answer. And she received the right answer. Every time she did not take the time to do that, she made the wrong decision.

I tested this after coming back home to my reality. The first couple of days, it worked fine. On the third day, I was too tired to get up early to meditate, and I went to work without doing it. I felt the negative effects right away. I felt out of place and less centered. I decided that I have to give meditation my total commitment if I wanted to succeed. It cannot happen without constant practice. It is like a muscle, you have to keep working it to make it stronger. Practice makes perfect. And when I need answers, I ask one question. I do not get the clear answer right away. I get it later in the day in other forms. I have to pay attention.

Before I finish meditating, I visualize. I see myself having a great day or I visualize where I want to be and what I want to accomplish. Throughout the day, I try to find quiet spots to do smaller versions of this visualization. It feels amazing and the feeling of having accomplished a goal and seeing yourself in it, is not only great, but it speeds up the process of getting it. I also use the end of a meditation to be grateful for the world and for everyone and everything I have in my life.

I realized that responding to my emotional stresses by eating junk food had the effect of shutting down communication with myself. Meditation helps open up communication. I realized that as soon as a voice was trying to come out because of stress or anxiety, I tried to shut it down. No wonder I had been feeling pulled in two directions for years.

Sometimes it is not easy to be still when you are stressed and anxious. I can repeat the words "relax" and "breathe" over and over, and sometimes it just does not happen. That is when doing something more active before meditating helps. It helps to release the stress physically and sweat it off. A great one-hour workout helps me to be more relaxed during my meditation and throughout the day. Now I also do active meditating. This means that between my workout and my quiet meditation session, I stretch while starting to meditate. I put on my waves music and focus on parts of my body I am stretching. It is nice.

I had been doing my meditation practice for three months, breathing mostly from my belly because I found that I had a difficult time breathing from the chest. I had to force it, and it felt like a huge weight on my chest. I went to see my acupuncturist for other things, and we talked about that feeling. It turns out that I really had blockage that inhibited my breathing from my upper chest, and this directly affected my lungs. My anxiety felt like I had twenty extra pounds of stress on my chest, and the fact that I was starting to have difficulty breathing made it worst, so I modified my breathing during my meditation to start from the chest and work down to the belly. It worked for me. The lesson here is to listen to the experienced people, and, most importantly, do what is right for you.

One more thing that needs to be noted is the importance of oxygen. Your body needs oxygen, and more than what you might breathe in normally on an average day. Take ten deep breaths three times a day. Breathe in, hold the breath for as long as you comfortably can and then breathe out; empty it all. Sometimes when you are stressed, you forget to breathe or breathe sporadically. That is not good. After these simple sessions, I feel great.

Chapter 10 Summaries

- ➤ Learn about different types of meditation. Choose one that is good for you.
- ➤ Practice meditation every day. Find some quiet time for yourself.
- ➤ Visualize what you want in life. See yourself already having it.
- ➤ Breathe. You need that oxygen!

Chapter 11: Treatments

The purpose that you wish to find in life, like a cure you seek,
is not going to fall from the sky....I believe purpose is something
for which one is responsible; it's not just divinely assigned.
MICHAEL J. FOX
An actor, a writer, and founder of
the **Michael J. Fox** Foundation for Parkinson's Research

There are all kinds of treatments out there that can help you. Some are more expensive than others. I have used a lot of them, so I am speaking from experience. In this chapter, I will not talk about cosmetic surgery. I am not saying I am for or against it; I just choose to focus on non-invasive surgical procedures, which sometimes can do the job just fine without the pain and damage of general anesthesia. The focus on non-invasive procedures also falls into the theme of this book, which is to have a connection between body and mind. I find that forcing your body into an aggressive surgery that changes something that your body and mind is not ready to let go of goes against the principle of this book.

ACUPUNCTURIST

First, let's talk about acupuncture. You can do plenty of research on the Internet about it, but here is my experience. It is important to find a professional acupuncturist. You have to feel good with whomever you choose; you have to feel a connection. I have used a few, and I never stayed more than twice with a person I did not feel good with. I have used acupuncture for many things, including body aches (knees, elbows, back, neck, headaches, and stomachaches), anxiety, and insomnia. The acupuncturist is able to tell me if my liver, kidneys, or spleen is not working properly, and is able to work on these areas and suggest foods or teas I should add or remove for a while to improve my health. Quinoa has a terrible effect on me. It is like a rock was trying to pass through my intestines. It can leave me up all night crying my eyes out. Once, I had it by accident. I was in a restaurant, and it was in a recipe and I did not notice it. I went to see my acupuncturist and within minutes the pain had passed. It is amazing.

When you find a good specialist, share it with the world. The good ones deserve to be known. I always do, and I am always happy when others have a great experience because of my referral.

OSTEOPATH

For your bones and joints, I would suggest a good osteopath. It took me a while to find a good one. How do you know if your osteopath is a good one? Well, you should go in with a problem, and you should leave with the pain gone. Just one session can do wonders. I referred a friend to mine, and she came to see me after her session. She had had a knot in the middle of her back for years and then it was gone. She could not believe it.

I use an osteopath for overall maintenance. I have issues with my knees and back. I rode horses when I was young and fell a lot, so my back was in bad shape and I had a lot of migraines. After a few sessions, I was feeling much better. Now I go every six or eight weeks for maintenance, and I love it. On a side note, if you have neck and back problems, make sure you have the best pillows and mattress. It is crucial.

CHIROPRACTOR

Before I went to an osteopath, I was seeing a chiropractor. A chiropractor cracks you all over to realign your bones and vertebrae to where they are supposed to be. I had an amazing man who treated me for years, and it helped a great deal. After a while, though, I got fed up with getting my neck cracked. I started feeling afraid he would break something, and I would end up paralyzed. Of course, nothing happened, but that is why I wanted something smoother and moved to the osteopath. I still recommend the chiropractor, and I still go for emergencies.

DETOXING

I am assuming that if you lost weight, you learned a bit about nutrition. You might have been on a very specific diet, hopefully a healthy one. Eight months before my wedding, I went to a gym that offered a lot of options to help me: nutritionist, personal trainer, as well as a spa and medispa on site. I met with a young lady who was passionate about health, nutrition, and training.

The first thing she suggested was that I do a detox. She found I was bloated, and felt a detox would help identify which foods I was intolerant to. The detox lasted ten days and included three days of fasting. Before you do any type of detox or fasting (or any big physical change in your diet or your exercise regimen) check with your doctor. Also, keep in mind that detox and fasting are NOT weight loss programs. They are meant to cleanse the system and make you feel good. I find it helps me to reconnect with my body and gives me an excuse to have two weeks as "me" time. During the fasting days (one weekend plus one day), I stay home, I write, I read, I take a bath, and I get massages. I force the world to back off for a while and let me have my "me" time. I accept no invitations during those ten days of detox. It is amazing. I always come out of that time re-energized and rejuvenated. People actually notice the difference in me. This works for me; it may not for you. You have to respect your body and do only what works for you.

I do a detox with each changing of the seasons. There are all kinds of detox regimens out there. My girlfriend does one that is more severe than mine that lasts three weeks. I could not do hers; it is too harsh for my taste. I like mine and she likes hers. Find one that works for you, and the first couple of times you do it, make sure it is supervised by a specialist.

The detox also helped me discover simpler foods and simpler tastes. It helped me to find my taste buds again without sauces and salts. My detox uses organic foods, and it is amazing. Through the detox, I also learned to eat smaller portions. I now eat more often—five or six times a day—but I eat smaller portions and I feel better for it. I still tend to have too big a meal at night, but I am working on that. The detox also helped me kick the diet soda habit. I used to have a lot of soda every day. Now I have maybe one a month. The detox is amazing; it puts you back into you. Where you belong. I have picked up good habits with it, such as no longer chewing gum (except on planes), chewing my food more slowly, not eating in front of the TV when I am alone, and focusing on the moment. And the bonus is, because you are removing all the toxins from your body, your skin looks amazing.

CELLULITE

At the same time, I wanted to improve the look of my skin, and I did not want it to sag because I was losing weight. Let's talk about cellulite and body contouring treatments. I have tried everything I could find. I am the perfect Guinea pig. I have tried Endermologie, Lumicell, VelaShape, mesotherapy, drainage massages, Accent, and Thermage. Now, no matter what treatment you try for cellulite, you need to know some things:

1. You need to eat healthy and do weight training. You need to build muscles.
2. Whatever treatment you do, you will have to maintain it. You cannot think that you will do fifteen treatments and *voilà!* you're done. Oh no, it is a commitment for life.
3. Your genetic predisposition to cellulite is important. The women in my family have lots of it. My sister is the healthiest person I know; she eats well, exercises, and even has her business in that industry, but she has cellulite. Muscle training and eating well alone won't get rid of it. You have to try some treatments.
4. It has been my experience that my body adjusts to the treatments, and I stopped improving with them. This is why I have tried so many.
5. Take home those before and after pictures and those measurements. I know it is not pleasant to look at, but I asked at the place where I was getting the treatments if I could take them home. You forget how you were. I look at my thighs today, and I am not that satisfied. I look at the pictures of my thighs six months ago and suddenly I am pretty darn happy.

Let's look in detail at some of the treatments. This is based on my experience alone and the reaction my body had to the various treatments. Your body may behave differently. What worked and what didn't work was based on me, and, most importantly, on how good I was with my exercise and nutrition.

1. The first real treatment I tried was Endermologie. It is the one where you wear a white suit, so it is a good place to start for those who are shy about being naked. At first it is twice a week. You should do a minimum of fifteen treatments. Of course, it depends what phase your cellulite is at. Cellulite can be at an early phase (Phase 1) to an advanced phase (Phase 4). Some parts of your body may be Phase 1 and others may be Phase 4. For me, Endermologie worked pretty well for a time. However, I was disappointed that I had to go back again and again. At that time, I was still naïve about the maintenance phase of the program. I did this treatment for about four years, on and off, through weight gain and loss. Then my body just stopped reacting to it, and I was wasting my money. I was ready to move on to the next treatment. By the way, for details on how the treatment works, don't hesitate to go online. There are plenty of sites on it. The treatment did not hurt, and I had no side effects. It is something like a deep massage, and you can resume activities right after.

2. Lumicell Touch. This is a massage much like Endermologie except it has an infrared light and is directly on the skin. For all technologies, you will start at a low frequency and then move up to stronger treatments. I did the treatment with a special cellulite oil and mixed it with a French technique called papier-rouler. Before the Lumicell treatment, a therapist manually rolls your skin to detach the fat layers then start the Lumicell treatment. I went twice a week for fifteen or so treatments. It did not hurt, but you have to make sure they don't increase the frequency too quickly because it may damage the skin. Of course, the person who takes care of you enhances the experience. If the therapist is dedicated, nice, and caring, you will have a great experience. I purposefully pick women for

this kind of treatment; I need someone who understands what I am going through. I loved the woman who took care of me, and the treatment worked. I kept going for almost three years. Every time I would gain weight and go on a losing weight regimen, I would add these treatments to the package. They do help your self-esteem because if you are like me, independently of the dress size if my skin is full of orange dimples I still don't feel better even if I lost a lot of weight. After those few years, I realized that it was not helping anymore. It was time to look for the next treatment. I decided on VelaShape (or VelaSmooth).

3. VelaShape is the newer version of VelaSmooth. When I read about it online, it suggested a once a week regimen. So when I went for Vela Smooth and I was told, however, that for better results, twice a week was recommended. So I did it twice a week for ten sessions. It really kicked off something that was not working anymore with Lumicell. I used it during my pre-wedding months of workouts and detox. With the combination of all that, I had amazing results. The before and after pictures are great. I was really happy. My only frustration was with the pain. If you are at Level 1 or 2, it is fine. But if you want results, you have to go to Level 3, and, in some areas, it is painful. I had to ask the therapist to move to other areas to give me a break. I did bring my iPod to try to focus on something else while she was "beating me up." I actually got a little aggressive during the treatments because of the pain and had to apologize a couple of times. The therapist, however, told me that some women give up after only three treatments because of the pain. So prepare yourself because the treatment happens directly to the skin using a special spray or cream. Each treatment is one hour (as are most cellulite

treatments). I felt these treatments got me ready for the wedding. I did a few after the wedding for maintenance, but their machine broke and I stopped going for a few months. Note that the cellulite comes back if you stop the treatments. I have since found a place with the newer machine (VelaShape), and with a wonderful woman therapist. I am back in treatment and still getting results. When I have a special event or am going to the beach on vacation, I add a couple of treatments in there. I still have some orange skin because of my genetic disposition, but I have to learn to live with it.

I can also share with you some research I did on food and cellulite. I did extensive research on the Internet, but I cannot guarantee that there is a correlation. I have no proof, but I think good foot cannot hurt. Here is the summary of food that may help reduce cellulite:

- Blueberries and blackberries
- Cherries
- Mangoes
- Oranges
- Strawberries and raspberries
- Cranberries
- Grapefruits
- Apples
- Spinach
- Tomatoes
- Bell peppers
- Carrots

Of course, everyone knows that refined or processed food and soda is bad for you, as is coffee and a diet high in animal protein and alcohol.

It is easy enough to follow. Now that I have lost the weight, I am counting on my weight training to help improve my orange dimpled look. By the way, localized weight training is great for your muscles, but keep in mind that your overall body fat needs to be at a healthy level.

One last note on cellulite, do a good scrub to remove dead skin. You can get one of those gloves and do it at home, but get a good quality glove so you don't damage your skin. You can also use a dry brush; this is a natural brush that can be used right on your dry skin before the shower. Or treat yourself to a professional body scrub—they feel nice. I've also used scrub shower creams or soaps that you can use in your shower. It is hard for me to tell you how often you should do it, as it depends on your skin. I would suggest a minimum of once a week. Some people do it every day, but I think that is a bit much. I do it twice a week.

BODY CONTOURING

I wanted to lose fat in very specific areas, and I wanted to see if those body contouring treatments helped. By the way, a few years ago, I had liposuction on my stomach, and it was, for me, a horrible decision. It hurt, it was disgusting the day after when all the bloody juices came out, it left marks on my lower abdomen, and I gained the weight back anyway. If you are not ready in your head to be forever thin, don't do it. Now back to non-surgical treatments.

1. First, I tried mesotherapy. This is a series of injections in fat areas that melts the fat away and then exits the body naturally. I found it painful, and I got no results. It was not for me.
2. The second thing I tried was Thermage. I tried it on my arms. It was also painful and delivered no results. I was

warned that Thermage works best as a skin tightening solution for the neck and face and is not the best treatment for arms. Well, they were right!

3. The next thing I tried was Accent. I tried Accent on my face and neck because I wanted to ensure that my weight loss did not make my neck or face skin sag. I have to say that I did enjoy the results. People told me I looked great. I also tried Accent on my stomach while doing the VelaSmooth. They suggested that both together gave great results. I did have great results. My stomach was definitely flatter than when I was doing Vela Smooth alone.

4. The next thing I want to try, but have not yet, is UltraShape. It claims to remove three to five centimeters after three treatments in a localized area. I would also love to test the percentage of fat in my body before and after those treatments. I will let you know how that goes on my web side.

CREAMS

Let's talk about skin tightening creams. I have tried Yves Rocher, Biotherm, Clarins, Nivea, and expensive spa creams. I think that they may help on a very superficial level. Truthfully, however, I have spent a ton of money on creams with no real proof they work. I think it is psychological for me. I feel that if I put on the cream after a good scrubbing then I am treating my body well. It makes me feel good. I also used cream on the day of the wedding because I was told it temporarily tightens the skin. So why not! I found, though, that my skin gets a little dry after using those creams for a while. What I do now is switch between normal hydrating cream and cellulite cream. I also slow down in winter with cellulite creams and focus mostly on hydrating my skin.

A LITTLE EXTRA HELP ON VACATION

I love cruises and our favorite company is Celebrity. On one of my cruises, I tried the Elemis detox treatment. They put electrodes on my arms, thighs, and stomach and they wrapped me in a seaweed wrap. I swear to God, I lost inches. I took three treatments over two weeks. I know I lost a lot of water, not fat, and it is not a permanent solution, but it is pretty cool when you are on a ship with fancy evening dresses and bathing suits! If they offered it in my town, I would do it before a big event.

So there you go. This is my take on fat reduction, skin tightening and cellulite therapies. I think it is important to take care of cellulite, but I think it is equally important to realize there are limitations to what today's technologies can do. You have to learn to love yourself just the way you are once you know you have done everything you can. I fear for those who go for extreme makeovers. They don't give their brain or heart and soul time to follow and God knows it does take a while for all the parts of you to catch up. So do treatments because they make you feel good in your heart and in your core self.

Chapter 11 Summaries

> - Consider using an acupuncturist, osteopath, and/or chiropractor.
> - Think about detoxing and nutrition.
> - Review cellulite and body contouring treatments.
> - Do these treatment slowly.

Chapter 12: I Don't Want to Be Where I Am. Living in the Now.

If you want to be happy, be.

LEO TOLSTOY
A Russian novelist

This chapter came to me one Sunday morning when I woke up feeling anxious. Normally working out and meditating would bring down my anxiety, but that morning I was insisting on finding out why I was so anxious. I think finding healthy tools to combat anxiety (instead of binging) is important, but finding the cause of anxiety is crucial. So I got up, made a pot of decaf coffee, and wrote in my diary. For about twenty or twenty-five minutes, I wrote about nothing of consequence. Then I started writing about how unhappy I was at work, about the fact that I felt I was not doing what I was meant to do, even if I didn't know what that was. Then I realized I sounded like a broken record. I had heard all that before. I zoomed back in time in fast mode through my memories and realized that I had never been happy where I was. Now in my private life, I am the happiest I have ever been in my entire life, but instead of focusing on that, I was focusing on how miserable I was at work. For the life of me, I could not believe that I had developed a pattern of being unhappy in my present.

If I went back in time, it was clear that in my youth I felt my life was hell and I was stuck. I survived by wishing for a better life. I dreamt of the day after high school when I would leave home. And, by God, I did move away, far, far away. But by then I was seventeen, and I had already created a pattern that I would have for many years to come. I was away from home, living in Ontario for a summer job and saving for college in the fall. But instead of embarking on the best summer of my life, I was anxious and sad. I was anxious at being away from home (yes, ironic isn't it!) and sad to be away from my friends. The letters I wrote that summer!

I started college that fall at a campus that was about one hour away from my family home. My mom was not happy to see me go, but I just could not stay there anymore. My parents tried to get my siblings and me to live together but I would have none of it. I did not care if I had to eat peanut butter sandwich every day; I would live away from my family. It was a great move on my part. I had to develop an identity for myself. My college years were rough; I had little money, I was insecure, and, yes, I dragged my pattern right along with me. I was in college and it should have been fun. I had good friends, and I made the volleyball team, but I was anxious. I created problems for myself with the teachers, the course work, classmates, and I focused on the negative. I found myself wishing to be somewhere else and not enjoying the moment.

After college, I did not know what I wanted to do, so I found a job on a ranch near Calgary, Alberta. I did not enjoy that either, but it didn't last long. I had to quit because of a thyroid problem. I went home. My grandmother died that summer and my sister got married. Things were happening, people were moving on, but I wasn't happy. I took a job as a live-in nanny for a family that had two children. I was twenty-one and had no clue what to do with my life and I had no money. That job was a welcome hiatus for a while. It was nice family, and I loved the two little girls that I was talking care of. But I grew restless. I was young and felt driven, but had no clue what I was driven toward. I felt dissatisfied with my present situation.

After three years as a nanny, I said to myself, "For the love of God, you can be and do better than this!" Now I think raising children is an important job. I was a nanny, on and off, from the age of thirteen until the age of twenty-five, and it is great work. But I felt I was meant for something else. So I left. I went to work in a company as a girl Friday, and found I loved the office environment. After a couple of years, I went back to university at night. I worked hard at that job for years. But all through those ten years or so, I was dissatisfied with the way I looked, my boyfriends, my job, and my performance at school. And I swear to god, I am realizing this now. In this light, it looks different.

After I'd finished my bachelor's degree, I moved to a new job where I stayed for fifteen years. During that time, I went back to school to get my master's degree and then my PMP certification (an important certification for a project manager - from PMI: Project Management Institute). With this job, I found I had plenty to complain about. I complained about the way the place was run; I complained about colleagues and bosses; I complained that I was not moving up the ladder fast enough. I was a project controlling officer for a couple of years, but I outgrew it and wanted to be a project manager. Then I outgrew that and wanted to be a director and then a vice-president. My dissatisfaction was very specific. I knew I could be more, personally, and I knew I could do a better job in the position I wanted than the person who was currently doing it. I ran into a lot of brick walls as I moved up. Some people were insecure about their jobs, so they blocked me; others were worried about losing a good project manager and wanted me to stay right where I was. That, to me, was faulty thinking. I was going to move up in the company with or without their help. If I was good then they should have helped me move up. In some cases, I had to go above my boss's head, one level, sometimes two, to be heard.

In my personal life, I used to have the same pattern. I complained about my family, complained when I was single, and complained about boyfriends because I had a pattern of finding bad boyfriends. All this dissatisfaction finally sent me into psychotherapy. With the help of my therapist, I got rid of that pattern of finding bad boyfriends, and I found my amazing pearl (my husband) among all the fake jewels.

Without realizing it at the time, I was for the first time starting to resolve negative patterns in my close relationships. I had started to realize that I deserved to be happy. The one place in my life I could not and cannot complain about is in my relationship with my husband. Everything about it is beautiful, romantic, and right. I was ready in my head and in my heart to live a happy life, and I opened the door to the amazing relationship I have now. Our wedding and amazing honeymoon were perfect. Of course, we talk about things we want to improve together, but I don't have any negative feelings about us. I don't daydream of being somewhere else. I feel I am right at home. The first month after we moved in together, I could not believe how well I slept. I had never in my life slept well with a man in my bed. Now, it felt great.

So that Sunday morning when I couldn't shake my anxiety and started to write about it, I found that I was once again complaining about work and how frustrated I felt being stuck in my job. The company was actually a good company, and my colleagues were fine. But I was still daydreaming about a better job, a better home, and more luxurious vacations. I wanted to live somewhere where there were no harsh winters. But that got me thinking. Once I had the new job, the condo in San Diego, and the first-class vacations, would I still be complaining and being dissatisfied?

This was a big *aha!* moment for me (yes, I do get them!). I realized I would continue to feel dissatisfied unless I cleared up my bad pattern. The problem was in me, not out there. If I was going to continue to act unhappy and dissatisfied, then life would make sure to give me plenty of reasons to continue to feel that way. Once I'd had that realization, I knew I had to do something about it. I had to get rid of the bad pattern.

It is important to separate bad dissatisfaction from good dissatisfaction. I have no doubt that the instincts in my youth that created my mechanism of escape were the right ones at the time. But they don't work in my current reality. Let's look at good dissatisfaction. When you feel in your gut that you can and should be more than you are, then your sense of being dissatisfied in your current situation is a good one. I made it to being a vice-president in a major firm and completing a master's degree because I was dissatisfied. Can you imagine how unhappy I must have been to take thirteen years of night school? I focused on one semester at a time. At first, I focused only on a bachelor's degree before I'd even thought of a master's degree.

Being dissatisfied is good. It gets you moving and gets you where you need to be. The bigger the dissatisfaction, the bigger the action needed to get you out of your situation. So look around you and pinpoint the areas where you feel unhappy. I don't mean just complaining, but being honest that you deserve a better boyfriend or a better career.

Did you ever have the feeling that you were in a relationship that did not suit you anymore? Did you, for months, feel an ache but didn't listen? Did you try to force it and see only the good in the other person? Did you think, "Can I see myself with this person twenty years from now?" Did that thought make you depressed? Then you had your answer. You just needed to face it.

Making a change as big as a relationship is not easy, especially if you have been together for many years. But from the moment you know it is over, don't drag it out. Take action. If it feels right in your heart, then it is the right thing to do even if it feels scary. I am now with the right man, and I am truly happy. My relationship with him is proof to me that life can be amazing and that I can be happy and truly satisfied. Because I made that big change, I now believe that it can happen with my career and my body image as well. If I solved my pattern of seeking out bad relationships then I can solve other bad patterns, too.

I do believe that I can be truly happy with my career and feel rewarded by it. I am not there yet, but I know that with patience, persistence, and consistent work, I can get anything I want. Before, when you made a list of what you are dissatisfied with, it may have discouraged you. Don't let it discourage you. Don't try to change everything at the same time. Pick one item on your list and get moving one small step at a time. When you will see the positive results, it will push you on to resolve other areas of your life that you are unhappy with.

I noticed that at the office, I had no desire to be anything else. By that I mean to grow into another role within the organization. That was new to me, after 15 years. I have never not wanted my boss's job. This meant that my next move was going to be outside of that office. I started with small steps, like writing this book.

Now let's talk about the bad pattern of being dissatisfied because that is who you believe you are. If your dissatisfaction is a habit that is linked to how people treat you, to how you see yourself negatively, to a negative perspective that leads you to complain about everything from burnt toast to the rain, then it is a pattern that you need to change because it is not serving you well. It is not helping you be happy, content, satisfied and rewarded with life. Being dissatisfied with work or with my body image is how I was. That is not how I want to be. I was so used to complaining that I did not know how to do anything else. That is why I believe that I did not remain at my goal weight for very long because I continued to have a negative body image and felt that I might as well complain about it for real and bring back the weight!

But life does answer. So why not ask the right questions? Change your pattern of dissatisfaction and things will change. I know this may sound like things I have said in other chapters, but there are multiple ways to look at and talk about something. Keep looking, keep listening, and one will click with you as it has with me.

Chapter 12 Summaries

- ➢ Make a list of what you are dissatisfied with.
- ➢ Start making a plan to change what you can.
- ➢ Be happy that you are dissatisfied. That is what gets you moving.
- ➢ Stop being negative about everything. Change the words to describe your situation. Ask the right questions that will get you to where you want to be.

Chapter 13: Forgiveness

When you hold resentment toward another, you are bound to that person or condition by an emotional link that is stronger than steel. Forgiveness is the only way to dissolve that link and get free.

CATHERINE PONDER
An American minister of the Unity Church
and author of books in the prosperity field

It took me a long time to understand the benefits of forgiveness. Some of it is still a mystery to me; however, this quotation from Catherine Ponder describes it as best as I can see.

I have already written about how I needed to apologize for some of the things I did to my brother. Forgiveness goes both ways. It is not just about you needing to forgive others but you needing to apologize to others whom you have wronged, ask for their forgiveness, and forgive yourself for having done wrong. Of course, you don't HAVE TO do anything. You can just sit there and pretend it is not a problem. It all depends on what you want to accomplish. If you feel stuck in time, and have a weight on your shoulders that prevents you from moving on or if you are fed up with feeling resentment and guilt, then you are ready to take action.

MAKE A LIST

Being ready to take action is a great place to be. In this instance, start by making a list. What unresolved issue do you feel is holding you back? Who is living rent-free in your head?

I noticed that sometimes my unconscious helps me find the answers. It comes out through daydreaming, writing in my journal, or monitoring my thoughts. It sometimes comes out in my dreams. If you have the same dream (or same type of dream) over and over, it means your unconscious is trying to tell you something. It is amazing to me how the human race does not do more research into dreams and discover how they could be used to discover our inner-workings. Freud had the right idea.

So let's get down to it. Make that list. List anyone or any event that you feel is stuck in your being and affecting you today. It does not matter if you want forgiveness or if you need to be forgiven. If you think of someone or an event and you have big feelings towards it, put it on the list. Sometimes it is easier to start by writing the event, before you get to the individual. It can be anything—a graduation, a wedding, an event where you were abused or fired. As far as people are concerned, it can be anyone—sibling, parent, uncle, cousin, friend, ex-partner.

WHY FORGIVE?

If you wrote about an event, you will eventually link it to an individual. Now you are looking at that list and suddenly you feel overwhelmed by feelings and think, "Why forgive? Why relive all these emotions?" The truth is that you are already reliving them every day in you sub-conscious. What you need to do is bring your feelings to the front of your mind; realize and accept that the feelings exist and then get rid of them forever. You need to know that you are doing it for you. It is a self-centered position, but that is not only okay, it is necessary.

Visualize what being stuck in the past does to your present. It is like having a permanent doorway open and some of your energy is lost through that doorway all the time because it takes energy to keep it open. If you have one doorway open for every person and every event that remains unresolved from your past, can you imagine all that energy being lost? Energy that you could use in your present to accomplish your current goals? This is why you need forgiveness. You need to regain your energy, your center and you need to live in the present and enjoy the present. You cannot do that if you keep losing all that energy through all those doorways.

As mentioned, I was never happy where I was because I was stuck in all other dimensions of my past. This meant I could never be fully present in my current reality. I believe that where you are today—with illness and problems and frustration—is because of those doorways and all that precious energy being lost. The great news is, you have now decided to take care of it.

Now, you don't have to tackle your entire list at once and forgive or offer an apology to everyone today. Take it step by step. I would suggest starting small; however, there is probably nothing small on that list if you have been carrying it around for years! So just pick one event or person to begin with. Write down everything you remember about the event or person. Write out all the feelings you felt at the time and what you are feeling today. This exercise can be done whether it is someone who wronged you or if you wronged someone. Write down everything that comes to mind. What effect is this lack of resolution having on your life today? What are the impacts of not resolving this? How long have you been carrying it around? How long will you choose to let this impact you in your future? What are the impacts of not resolving this? What are you willing to do to resolve this problem? What actions do you need to take that will close that doorway for good? Are you willing to forgive or apologize? You need to be honest when you answer all these questions:

that is important. Let all the emotions go through you—sadness, anger, frustration, and feeling powerless, victimized or annoyed. Whatever you feel is okay. If, you feel after all that, you are not ready to move forward with the event or person you picked, choose another. Keep in mind, that you are doing it for you. You want to free yourself. This helps when, for example, you are looking at forgiving someone who abused you (physically, psychologically, or sexually). It makes it easier if you stay focused on you. When I did not understand the concept of forgiveness, I thought, "Why on earth would I forgive him? He does not deserve it." But I deserved it. And you do. You deserve it for yourself.

ESTABLISH WHAT IS SUCCESS FOR YOU

The next step is to decide if you need to complete this process in person. Some people write a letter to the person and burn it, and they find that that is enough. You will know pretty fast if that is enough. In some cases, writing is good; in other cases, you need to see the person. I find that most of the time, and if the person is alive, I need to see him or her. I need to feel it. If you've decided to go to that meeting, it is important to be prepared. You need to have clear expectations. You cannot control or guess how the other person is going to react. Frankly, it does not matter. You are there for you. You are there to forgive or to apologize. How you do it is very personal. How you approach the person is up to you. There are many ways that will work. But ask yourself if you are entering this get together from a place of anger. Do you need an explanation? Some do—some want to know, "Why me?" You will also not approach everyone the same way. It depends on who they are and what they did, but, mostly, it depends on how you feel about the person. As an example, you may want to meet someone who abused you. You'll find that a lot of people are not in touch with their emotions and will be uncomfortable with the discussion. The person you approach may turn aggressive or evasive, saying you imagined the whole thing or invited it by your actions. You may hear all kinds of things. That is why you have to detach yourself from the reaction. How the person you approach reacts is not your problem.

I have gone through this process a few times. One time, I approached a person who had been psychologically, verbally, and physically abusive (not sexually) toward me. He pretty much denied the whole thing. The events had happened years before, and he seemed to have re-created events to suit his behavior and made himself look okay. He said that he acted that way because it was for best for me, that he wanted to turn me into a great adult, that it was what I needed, and that he was being supportive in his own way. Wow, I could not believe what I heard. He was so stuck in his way of looking at things, that no matter how much I tried, he could not understand my side of things and listen to how I had lived through those events and felt at the time. He was clearly closed down and did not want to get in touch with any feelings about it. He was like a robot, reciting something from a book. So at that point, I did what I came to do. I said what I wanted to say totally for my own benefit, and two weeks before his death, I told him I forgave him. In a way, I was lucky. I was able to forgive him before he passed away, and now I am free. I feel it: it is one less weight on my shoulders and that door is closed.

Again, preparing yourself is the key to success. Define, for yourself, what a successful meeting would be for you. What are your parameters? There is a woman in my life that I am not particularly fond of. She is a relative, and there is always some event that we both attend. Almost every time, she will corner me to tell me something she wants to get off her chest. It is never done in private. There are always people we know in the same room, and she will aggressively tell me in front of them, what I did or said that hurt her or about rumors that she heard of me talking about her. Although I appreciate her need to clear the air, she made some mistakes in her approach.

> ➤ She should have given me fair notice that she wanted to discuss this matter before the event so I could prepare myself.
> ➤ She did it in front of people we know. Do not do that. The person confronting you can try to gather those people to their cause against you. You don't need that. With that said, I prefer to meet in public, such as a restaurant or a café, with strangers around because I don't want to meet alone and in private with the person. When I need extra support, I ask someone I care for to be at another table in case I need them.
> ➤ Approaching someone like this will usually result in a complete shut down. I told her it was not the time or place and closed the discussion. Not only did she not get closure, but now I think she is an annoying idiot and I like her even less. I will not be open to further discussions on the matter in the future.

She clearly was not prepared for our meeting. She started from a place of impulse and strong unresolved feelings. She had not identified for herself what would be the criteria for success.

Have your in-person meeting when you feel ready. There is no reason to force things. If you do, you may find that the meeting will flop and you will feel worse. I still have my list, and when I feel the need, I approach one person on my list. There are some that I am nowhere near ready to approach and that is okay. I will when I am ready.

It is the same process when you feel you need to apologize to people. Prepare yourself, and prepare your success parameters. The person you approach may not forgive you— ever. So, again, you have to do what is right for you and your conscience. I apologized to my brother, and I included him in the most important event in my life, my wedding. I love him, I respect him, and I am proud of him. My criteria for success were to apologize, tell him I love him, and include him in my life. The rest was not up to me, so I let go of it. He told me we were good, and he had no bad feelings. I was lucky, but it may not turn out so well. The other person's reaction cannot be part of your success criteria. You cannot force someone to forgive you. But if you accomplish your goal, you can close another door and move on.

In the cases where you need to apologize to someone for your wrong behavior, you will also need to forgive yourself. It is necessary. We are all human and we all do things we are not proud of. Even if you apologize and the person forgives you, you may still not feel satisfied. That is because you feel bad and guilty about how you behaved. You need to forgive yourself. It is important in order to let the situation go. Go through the same process of writing down the events, writing down your feelings, and why you think you behaved the way you did. Learn from that experience, forgive, and move on.

In the case of my brother, I wanted a friendship with him. However, in most cases, you don't want a relationship with the person you are meeting. Because you chose to forgive someone who wronged you does not mean you have to see them on a regular basis. You do not. You never need to see them or talk to them again. That was new to me. I thought I needed to have a relationship with those I forgave. Chances are the people you have met with and forgave are not people you would hang out with anyway. They have different values.

The great news is that as an adult, you can choose who to have in your immediate circle of friends and acquaintances.

DID IT WORK?

You know forgiveness or apologizing worked when you feel relaxed, when you feel a weight has been lifted from your shoulders, or when that person is no longer in your head. Listen to yourself. I can be impulsive and emotional and there were times when I did not do this right. I could feel it was not resolved. There were times when I wrote a letter, burnt it, and yet felt the feelings were still there. Put the person or event back on the list and deal with it later, when you are ready.

Take it easy and take it one step at a time. There is no way around this process if you want to move forward, and it needs to be done right. It is the same as going on a quickie diet that will help you lose twenty pounds in one month and regain it (and more) two months later, and having to start all over again with a diet that begins slowly from the head and heart so you will never regain the weight. Being and feeling free: that is what it is all about.

Chapter 13 Summaries

➤ Make a list.
➤ Should you meet face to face or not?
➤ Prepare for your meeting.
➤ What are your criterias for success?
➤ What are your expectations?
➤ Be patient. Do it when you are ready and do it right.

Chapter 14: It's Okay If You Can't See It—Have Faith

Just one mental shift—focusing on the abundance of your environment—switches your psychological settings so that your life automatically improves in many areas you may think are unrelated. This is essentially a leap from fear to faith.

Martha Beck
An American sociologist, therapist,
life coach, and best-selling author

I love the song, "I Surrender All." The version I love the most is the one by Faith Hill I heard on the Oprah Show. I get goose bumps. During that show, Oprah talked about how she came to act in the Color Purple. It totally illustrates what this chapter is all about. Sometimes, you do not have all the answers. You may not know how you are going to get to where you want to be. You may feel the hole is too big to get out of. The weight on your shoulders may be so heavy that you just don't know how to go on. This is not a chapter about religion; it is a chapter about faith. It is a chapter about thinking that life is bigger than just little old you. The minister at my wedding interviewed my future husband and me to prepare what she would say during the ceremony. She described each of us, and for me, she said, "She believes in the Universe."

SMALL STEPS

The best way to deal with a huge and daunting task is to start small. Make your plan. See where you are at and where you want to be. Then do one little thing every day to move forward. That is important. You will gain momentum. When I was in my early twenties, I was depressed. I had gone through a horrible and destructive experience while in college and I barely finished it. I felt horrible, and all my big dreams after high school not only seemed unattainable, but I wondered how I would get through the day! However, no matter how low I felt, I always had this sense that I was meant to be more than what I was at the time. I had this voice inside of me that said, "You can get out of this." It was my light at the end of a very long tunnel. I had faith in something bigger than my own self. I did not always listen. Sometimes I would go on being and feeling down for weeks, not knowing how to get out of it, and making the wrong choices for me. I wish I knew then what I know now. But I took small, small steps, one day at a time. I made a list of what made me feel good, and I would force myself to do one of them every day. At that time, medicine for anxiety and depression was not as advanced as it is today, and I was not in therapy. My first goal was to make myself feel better about life. Slowly, I got better. I also accepted that it would take me a little while to get to my next goal and gave myself a break. I did not give up on my goals; I realigned my plans so I could get there more slowly. My mind and body were not ready to jump and take massive action. I took it slower and as I got mentally healthier, I took bigger leaps. Everyone knows that winter will change into spring and summer, you know that night turns into day. I was going through winter at that time, and my little actions took me towards spring.

FAITH, YES. BUT GET ORGANIZED

I write about unwavering faith in myself as if I had it all together and I was a self-assured woman. God, no. I was riddled with doubts. I had people around me who reinforced my low self-esteem and made fun of my dreams and goals. Slowly, I started to separate myself from those people. That was one of my first step. I did not do it all at once. I did it slowly but surely. Even today, I don't always listen to my intuition and that always ends up harming me in some way. When I have doubts about my actions, and when I question everything, I turn to faith. At some point, I have to stop saying, "What if?" and be quiet and silent and just listen and believe. There are many times in my life when I was in a deadlock and somehow got out of it. I know I can eventually attain my goals.

I believe that the combination of having unwavering faith with my ability to organize and plan got me to where I am today. I strongly believe that one without the other will not work. I could sit around all day and hope for things to happen, but that will get me nowhere. Action is needed—big or small. And this action needs to be flexible. When I started writing this book, I was inspired and wrote plenty during the two weeks I was in Hawaii. When I got home, there were times when I had no inspiration and I would not write at all for weeks. But I felt that even if I was disappointed and I wanted to get the book out, I could not force it. So I modified my plan and worked on other things while I waited for inspiration. I read up on how to get published, how to create a web site, how to find a designer for my book cover. I thought about what I wanted for my book cover and did all kinds of research on the Internet. I also used all the tools I've written about in this book and practiced them again and again. Eventually, I would get the urge to write and I might write three chapters in one weekend. But during all that time, I knew I was fine. I knew I would get it done because I had faith.

LOOK AT THE PAST

Sometimes when I have doubts about what to do next, I go back to my past. I try to remember the times when I had hardships and how I got past them. If there is some specific hardship, I go through my memory banks to see if I have lived through it before. I found it amazing how much stuff I had forgotten, and a lot of the time, I would discover I'd gone through something similar before. Looking at past events reinforces how much of a role faith had in my choices. Thinking back, I am amazed how many times the right cards fell into place and the Universe answered. I have so many examples of that happening in my life. Every time, I managed to survive through a mix of faith and taking some form of action. It is like a domino effect. One thing leads you to the next step and the next step.

Looking back buffers me from my doubts of today. Every time I did something new or when I reached for a bigger goal, I went through periods of doubt. Looking back on how I succeeded makes me feel secure; I know that I will succeed, although not always in the way I think I will. Getting organized and planning your next steps is great but at some point you have to stop planning and jump; do it and have faith.

IS THIS THE RIGHT GOAL?

There are times when my life went in a completely different direction than what I had expected when I set a goal. You can plan and organize all you want, but the Universe has a say in it too. This is the faith part. And this is why it is important to be flexible and readjust your goals according to the new direction your life is taking. For example, I always wanted to win the lottery. Sometimes, I would wish for the big prize, millions of dollars, and sometimes I just wanted $50,000 to make my life easier. But somewhere, deep in my soul, I didn't believe I would ever win. Winning would be too easy. Having millions in my bank account tomorrow morning would stop my urge to be more and do more. I would completely miss out on becoming the woman I am meant to be. I would not finish this book, have a website, do conferences, or help people. I had discovered a belief and that was amazing—an *aha!*

moment. Knowing this, what am I going to do? Readjust my goal. Forget the lottery. I decided to make my own success, financial or otherwise. I closed another doorway. As long as I believed I could win the lottery and bought tickets, I was wasting energy. Then I accepted my belief that it was not my way, and I could focus on taking massive actions towards my goals.

Writing this chapter was a pleasure. It forced me to get out of my logical and analytical side and reconnect with the unknown, and be okay with that unknown. I used to be so uncomfortable that it would make me anxious. Now, most of the time, I welcome it. I know life will answer at the proper time. But don't forget that life needs some help and action is needed to reach the place you want to be at. Have some quiet time for yourself. Meditate or just be alone, quiet. Stay still, otherwise you might miss the answer.

Chapter 14 Summaries

- ➤ What is faith for you?
- ➤ Combine your faith with a plan.
- ➤ See how you succeeded in the past.

Chapter 15: Don't Lose Your Focus after a Big Event, and Don't Let Day-To-Day Life and its Problems Distract You from Your Goals

If you don't like something, change it. If you can't change it, change your attitude.

MAYA ANGELOU
An American author and poet

Well, I am back at work and my old habits are trying to come back. I am sticking to my meditation. I firmly believe that it will make a difference. I need to remain centered at all cost. But I am eating junk food again. I have to put a stop to that now, period.

I wrote this soon after I came back to work after the honeymoon. It was a nice goal, but eleven months later, I had fallen back into old patterns. I let daily life's problems get the best of me. I slowly lost sight of my goals. They were stuck in the background. I forgot to keep an eye on my thoughts and patterns. I got caught up with work and the stresses of daily life. Here I am telling you what to do and I don't have it all together myself. Well, that is reality; I am going through this the same as you are.

When you are fed up with your current circumstances and you read a book like this, you get all pumped up and you make your lists and follow through. As soon as it is better or close to what you were aiming for, you lose the urge to continue. You stop doing the training or the meditation or the listening to your thoughts or fixing your bad patterns. Whether you geared up for a big event or reached a goal, once it is over and completed and you've felt the success, you will then feel down, and it will make it hard for you to keep going.

WHAT'S NEXT?

My problem was that I did it all for a big event, the wedding. I did not follow all the suggestions that I have put in this book consistently. I focused only on the outside and not the inside. I lost my focus when the big event was over and when the daily stresses of life got in the way. My husband and I worked on our wedding for fifteen months. I have worked on myself for over forty years, but for eight months, I worked intensively. I had better nutrition, harder training, more detoxing. We had the wedding, and it exceeded our expectations. We had the honeymoon of our dreams. When we came back, we saw the pictures of the wedding and we looked amazing. I was amazed at how smiley and relaxed I looked before the wedding. Never in my life have I ever been like that (the anxious type remember?). I could not believe the way I looked; I really was a princess that day. When I came back to work, a colleague asked if I felt depressed now that it was over. I was totally taken by surprise with the question. It had never occurred to me that I would. But she was right. I was not depressed, but I had to give myself some time to "grieve" the loss of that magic event that would never come back. I found I had tears in my eyes when I looked at the pictures. The love between my husband and I, the love we felt from our guests, the pure joy and happiness that is evident on our faces and those of our guests was truly magical, and I thought, "Oh, my God! What can come after that? What can top that?"

SLIPPERY SLOPE

When I came back to work after the honeymoon, people were amazed at how peaceful and glowing I looked. Some said they had never seen me so relaxed, and I have been there for fifteen years. Suddenly, I found I was afraid to lose the good feelings and sense of well-being that I had acquired at the wedding and during the honeymoon. What do you think started happening? I started slowly losing it and regaining the weight. Within one week, six days in fact, I had a small binging moment. After all this work, losing those pounds, looking amazing! My younger self could not handle my amazing success, and that part of me was hell bent on screwing it up. Because I had added daily meditation to my mourning routine, I managed to stay calm through lunch, but as soon as afternoon hit, the voices started, "Wouldn't a chocolate bar (or four) taste great right about now?" Because of a lack of time, sometimes I chose to meditate rather than work out. That did not help the situation. I realized I needed both. But I was slowly but surely sliding back into a cycle I'd swore I wouldn't ever fall into again. I thought that I would have to find another goal that was worthy of eating well, exercising regularly, and maintaining my weight.

YOU ARE ENOUGH

Then I realized that my goal could not be an external goal. I had to overcome my bad relationship with food. I had to solve my dilemma once and for all. The goal became to not eat junk food as an outlet for an emotional reaction. It was not a small goal. I daydreamed about the times when I would be happy and comfortable in my body. Then a sentence said many times by Oprah just popped into my head: "You are enough." It kept popping up in my head. I am enough. I am enough to justify the hard workouts and the healthy food. I didn't need an external event to justify to myself that I am worth it. I can look and feel as amazing as the day I got married anytime I choose. It is my choice, and any pressure I feel is brought on by only one person, me. I am not saying to heck with it, or that life is too short and I will live it however I want. What I am saying is that you need to tell yourself

1. I am worth it and I am enough. I am a great enough reason to want to look and feel amazing. I don't have to create an event or an external goal to reach my best self. I can do it now. I can decide right now that today, this afternoon, this hour is a time when I am and I feel amazing. I look amazing because I am worth it. Writing down your affirmation will help alleviate your stress. Don't do it for any other reasons than because of the way it makes you feel about yourself and the way you look. Internalize it: "It is mine and the reason is me." You don't have to prove anything to anyone and when you don't do what's best for yourself, you hurt only one person, you.

2. I want to keep on feeling this way. I want exercise because I love the feeling of well-being and pride and connection I have with my body. I want to eat healthy because now that I learn more and more about the human body, I want to treat it—and treat me—better. I want to feed me in a way that my body will work optimally.

3. I want to treat myself with respect because it feels amazing. Being able to fit into your jeans comfortably and hearing your husband sat that you look great feels nice, but I want to feel good regardless of these external merits. I want to treat myself with respect.

4. I want to be 100% responsible and 100% committed to myself. When I saw the pictures of the wedding after the honeymoon, I was in awe of how I looked. But I was also

thinking, "Oh, my God! I want to keep looking like that but it's too much work (limiting belief)." That is pure laziness talking and envy. I envy people who can eat whatever they want and still not gain weight. I get angry and I get lazy; I put myself into a mindset that I deserve a treat. I deserve that chocolate and I deserve not to work out today. But that treat is really a punishment. Every time I don't work out when I had planned to or when I eat junk food, I mistreat the one person I should love the most. I mean, who else are you going to spend your whole life with but you? I need to choose. I need to take 100% responsibility for my choices and actions. I need to stop sitting on the fence. Do I want to be average or great? I can't have my cake and eat it, too. I can't feel amazing after eating junk food. It is a choice. Therefore, no cake and a good work out. My biggest problem when I got back from the trip was that I would give myself excuses for cheating. And that is inexcusable! Every time you make yourself a promise and then break it, you hurt yourself. You give up on yourself and then hate yourself. Sometimes I find that I am better at keeping my promises to others than myself. But am I less worthy than they are? That is a big "No!"

I believe that it takes hard and consistent work for me to maintain my weight. Therefore, I have two choices: change that belief or accept it. Let's say I accept it. That means that I have to stop envying those who don't need to work at it to maintain their weight. I need to keep in mind that I have big goals. I don't want to be average. I want to be great. That takes work, period. Stop trying to get by with the minimum of work. Set your mind straight. Anything worth having is worth working for. I have big dreams and goals, and I don't mind hard, consistent work. Some people tell me I am too demanding with myself. But, as I said before, don't break a promise you made to yourself. What this means is be sure to build into your plan some space for change and adjustments.

You will have some fall backs. Leave some space where you can relax and have drinks with friends, romantic dinners in restaurants, and birthday cake at parties without labeling it as failure. Sometimes you will be on a trip and there will be nothing to eat except unhealthy food. Give yourself a break. However, if you planned to go to the gym after work, don't let friends distract you from your goal. If you do have the not-so-healthy food, put your secondary plan in motion and get back on track as soon as you are able. Don't beat yourself up; it is unnecessary and hurtful.

Does it get easier? Life does not get easier but how you deal with it can. Just remember that the more you grow, the more you will be challenged. I used to wait for the day when I could say, "Now I can sit down and relax because I have conquered my fears and my demons and I have reached my goals and my dreams." I know now that that day will never come. People thrive on more—getting more and being more. Granted, it is not relaxing, and it is sometimes downright exhausting, but at the same time, it is exciting and uplifting. Let's take some examples. After highschool, I wanted to get out of my parents' house and go to college. I did that. At twenty-two, I wanted to stop studying and get a job. I did that. At twenty-five, I wanted to get an office job because those people with access cards attached to their hips with pictures on them looked important and part of a secret group. I wanted in. I did that. From that point on, I was trapped. I am an achiever and fundamentally envious of what I can have that I do not. I am the perfect candidate for the office world because bosses can easily take advantage of someone like me. Work work work. I am a person with a tremendous desire to move up the corporate ladder. Titles I got in my job were great but only for a time, and then I worked towards something else. At my first office job, I was replacing someone on vacation and they kept me on. Give me anything. I was lucky that my first boss was a career woman. She encouraged me to be and do more. I looked up to her. So very soon, I wanted more. My boss moved away, and a woman replaced her and that did not go well with me. What I needed in a boss was someone who would drive me to do and be more, a boss who was smarter and quicker than I was and someone who respected me. I needed a boss to be a mentor to me. Otherwise, it wouldn't work out. I have to say that anytime I got less than that, I had problems and ended up leaving.

Sometimes you need to change companies to change your role. At some companies, people will always see you in your current role and unless you leave, you will stay stuck there. I changed companies and I changed my role. I am stubborn when I want to be! The thing with me is I have my self–doubts, but I also have a huge drive and an underlying belief that I can do it. That mix slowed down my progress, but I advanced anyway.

After being a secretary, I became an assistant estimator in a construction company. I had only a junior college degree so what I could be was limited. I decided to go back to university and slowly, at night, I obtained my bachelor's degree. The mix of working and studying made me want even more because I began to know more. After being an assistant estimator, I went on to manage a small construction office. I had by then started therapy, and this also pushed me to be more. If at any given time I felt that the atmosphere and respect in an office was deficient, I left. After I finished my bachelor's degree, I was hired as a project coordinator in the company I am now with. My boss encouraged me to do my masters' degree right away. So I went back to school at night and got that degree. At work, I saw other positions, higher than mine, that I wanted to have. You have no idea how much I had to fight to get them. People kept blocking me. I was too young, too in-experienced, but, mostly, I was too good at what I was doing and nobody wanted me elsewhere. I am not blowing my own horn.

Supervisors have told me that they wanted me to stay in my job as a project coordinator because they needed me. But I became a project manager and, after a few years, I wanted to advance higher and ran into the same problems. The same thing happened when I became a director and then vice-president. There are times when it took years to get into a new role. I had to learn to be patient and to go to the right people to get it done. Thankfully, I ran into some good supervisors. They saw my potential and helped me achieve different levels of success.

In all these career moves, my level of anxiety never lowered. Every time I did something new, the stress was huge. Why? Because I was out of my comfort zone. Then I began to enter a new phase. I was tired of the corporate world. I was beginning to be in a place where I was enjoying life more. I wanted to use my creativity—something that I had put away years ago. I wanted a career that made me happy to get up in the morning. I did no longer wanted to stress over the office rat race.

So I still had drive, and I still had the urge to do more, but I didn't want to go up the corporate ladder anymore. I wanted to develop some ideas I had. I wanted to start a web site, write a book, and give some conferences. I did not know where to start, so I started with this book. I figured a journey of a thousand steps started with the first step.

So how can it get easier if you keep on wanting to improve and be more? People need to grow, consistently. But even growth has some downtime. Use this downtime to reassess your position, assimilate new data, see where you want to be and how you are going to get there. Remember my meditation teacher in Maui who had said that his sister had told him that for the last three months of the pregnancy there was nothing to do but to let it happen. The same thing can be said here. Let things settle. It can last weeks or months. I don't like those times much, but they are necessary. This is the unknown phase I was referring to in the last chapter. I was not anxious about it but very frustrated. It is annoying to know that I was ready for something else, but not quite ready to jump into it. You will move on to the next stage, but only when life says you are ready, not when you say you are. The stages of life are like butterflies. The time in the cocoon is crucial and necessary. You cannot bypass that period. Well, the same thing is true for humans. If you don't respect your transition stage and do what is necessary while you are in that stage, then you will not be ready for the next stage. And don't let others decide when your quiet stage is over, either. How many examples are there of humans who became too rich and too famous too soon and then fell? Some died; some disappeared to a quiet place. Why do so many lottery winners lose their winnings after a short time? They bypassed the cocoon stage altogether.

As you grow, you learn. As you gather momentum, you are able to take on bigger and bigger challenges. You feel more secure and more self-assured, and your belief in yourself grows and grows. So even if life keeps throwing challenges at you, you are better equipped to handle them. But you will get to where you want to go. And everything in this book and in the supplementary reading will help you get there.

So how do you not lose your focus after a big event? How do you not let life's daily problems take over? Well, first and foremost, make yourself a priority. You matter most in your own life. You cannot help others if you are not at your best. It is not selfish. You are the one person you will spend all your life with, so you deserve your "me" time. The next step is to develop great beliefs, habits, and patterns. They will help you stay on track even when daily life gets in the way. Make a list of what is important to you. Take action every day and do one thing—big or small. Do not let the day end without some form of action. Momentum will help you get back on track.

After a big event, how long will you give yourself before you bring up the stop sign and say, "Enough"? My stop sign is at five pounds. If I had gained five pounds then I need to put everything in motion to lose it again. Another stop sign was three days: never more than three days without exercise. It is good to have these stop signs, but why let yourself gain five pounds or take three days off in the first place? Take a moment to consider what was going on in your life that made you eat bad food or slow down on working out. In order to follow your new you, it is important to not just to look at the number on the scale. You need to look inward. Take a moment every night before bedtime to see if you had a great day, as per your definition. If you did not have a great day, why not? Your goal is not the weight number but the well-being you want to feel every day about yourself.

Because I started binging again so soon after I came back from the honeymoon, it was obvious I had not resolved my emotional eating issue. This had to become my top priority; otherwise, I was going to struggle for the rest of my life. And struggling takes a lot of energy. Really, it's exhausting! And I really wanted to use that energy elsewhere. I wanted to build something great that would require all my focus.

You need to look for the thing that is sabotaging your efforts to keep the weight off the most. Look for the thing that is preventing you from having a healthy relationship with food and attack it full on. If you don't conquer it, you are wasting your time. Sometimes it may be a deep psychological issue, and if this is the case, get help. Face it. But sometimes you may just need to take massive action, take full responsibility for yourself, and make a choice. You are where you are today because of the choices you made. Yes, external events, bad ones and even horrible ones, have occurred in your life. No doubt about it. But how are you going to act now? How are you going to react to those events today? That is what is important. Why carry around pain and anxiety from events that occurred in your youth? The only reason is because you choose to. It is your choice to let those events affect your life today. Is it worth it? Is it serving you well? Is it helping you become who you want to be? I am guessing not! Well what are you going to do about it? It takes courage to face that. Do it, one step and one day at a time. But do it. Take action.

I had entered a pattern of excuses; I told myself that I ate because of this or because of that. And because I had reasons to justify my behavior, I was okay. But I wasn't! I needed to break that pattern. It may have been helped me once, as a survival mechanism, but now it was hindering my happiness and progress.

To help break the pattern, I set up a series of questions and actions that I immediately do. This is what works for me, and you might find it helpful as well.

1. Stop, breathe, listen, and ask why?

2. Just don't do it. Don't reach for the food. Give yourself a timeframe—fifteen, thirty minutes or one hour. Drink water during that time. If you still desperately need the food, then go for it, but eat consciously. Don't disappear into no man's land. Have one treat. Not ten.

3. Can you change your focus? If you feel bored, rejected, and/or anxious, and your normal pattern is to reach for food, well, try something else. And then try something else again and again and again and again until something else fills that need. Review the chapter on changing patterns and take action.

4. Learn what your triggers are and prevent them. I leave the house every morning in a state of relaxation after my meditation. By the time noon hits, however, I have worked myself into a frenzy of stress and frustration. I feel like I have no other way out but binging. The key is to stop the pattern before it starts. Make sure you don't get to the point of needing the food. Once you become conscious of your triggers and patterns, it is quite amazing to observe yourself. As soon as you identify a trigger, stop it or turn it around. For example, if you know that watching TV makes you eat, then don't turn the TV on or exercise in front of it.

5. Ask yourself, why your younger self is making so much noise. What happened lately? Write down your thoughts in your journal. Your younger self may feel wounded and is trying to communicate. Listen, love, hug, and forgive.

6. Be grateful. Every time you are about to lose it and binge, think of it as an opportunity given to you to solve this issue once and for all. Instead of focusing on the problems, focus on the solutions outlined in this book and take action.

If setting a regular weight goal helps you stay on track, then go ahead. Find events or create events throughout the year where you want to look your best and plan accordingly. But it is crucial that you don't do it for others. You have to do it for yourself, and you need to do it because it makes you feel good. I vowed that I would try on my wedding dress once a year. I chose that event because it makes me feel great and returns me to a magical moment in my life. Going on vacation is also a good event for when you want to look your best. You could pick family events but those can be dangerous if you find that they are filled with all kinds of emotions. So be careful with those. I created an event by booking a photo shoot four months after my wedding with our wedding photographer. I wanted to do it for myself; I wanted to see through his lens that I was beautiful. I had a great time, and I had a magazine made with the best fifty pictures. It is a great gift that I gave myself.

After a big milestone or a big event is over, you will probably go through a down time. Either you will feel you have reached the top so you can stop working hard or you will be sad that after so many months of work, your one day is gone. It is okay to feel this way. All feelings are okay. You have to accept the different stages of a big event: elation, pride, happiness, sadness, and letting go. Be ready to let it go. Embrace the memories and move on. Pick your next target and work towards it. Keep on working on improving your relationship with food. This does get easier.

As you listen more, as you pay more attention to your needs, as you improve your beliefs and patterns, you will feel better about yourself and you will love the feeling of respect you give yourself.

Binging was one way I had to shut myself off from myself, not listen to myself, not listen to my pain. How can you feel self-love and self-respect if you are not even willing to listen to yourself? Techniques such as giving yourself thirty minutes or one hour before you jump into the junk food gives you time to ask yourself some key questions and open a dialogue with yourself. I don't believe in putting a Band-Aid on a problem. You have to get to the bottom of things, and solve them one problem at a time.

Don't forget to write in your journal. You may feel an overload of information sometimes and writing things down helps you to get some perspective.

Start acting *as-if*. Don't ignore problems, but start acting as if you were ready to listen and solve them one at a time. Don't act anymore like the person who gives up, who thinks it's too hard, or who has an "I can't" attitude. Act as if you had already reached your goals and been successful for years. And before you know it, your real life will catch up to the new you—to your new story.

Chapter 15 Summaries

➢ The big event is over. What's next?
➢ Do not let the daily stresses of life steer you away from your goals.
➢ Why are you enough? Make a list.
➢ Discover how to stop the binging ritual.
➢ Keep working on getting better beliefs and patterns.

Conclusion

"The world 'out there' won't change until the world 'in here' does."
DEEPAK CHOPRA
A medical doctor, public speaker, and writer on
subjects such as spirituality, Ayurveda, and mind-body medicine.

I don't have it all together. Based on what I had in my life and who I was five years ago, I have some of it together. Based on the new challenges, the new people, and the new events in my life now, I'm not even close to having it all together. But I am much better equipped to deal with it. I am still learning, adjusting, growing, and changing. They say that the one consistent thing in life is change. They are right!

What does a conclusion mean in a book like this? It means that searching to improve ourselves never ends. Every day, month, and year, there is something else to improve or change. And that is great news.

What have I learned by listening to myself and writing this book? I would never lose weight permanently and have a healthy relationship with food until I resolved why I gained it in the first place. In order to do that, I had to learn quite a bit more about myself and look deep into things I had been burying. I did all the exercises in this book and answered all the questions. And I didn't do them just once; I did them again and again. Because who I was and who any of us are in March of any given year and who you are in December will be different. Everyone changes, grows, and falls back a little. A part of yourself that was inaccessible six months ago may open up to you in the days or weeks to come.

If you have followed through the chapters in this book, do you find that you are now keeping an eye on your thoughts? Do those thoughts reflect who you want to be and not who you were? Keep focusing on them and keep improving them. As you begin to change a habit, you may find you need to focus on it every day. After a while, once it is well ingrained into your being, you may need to check up on it only every once in a while. But never think that you will never have to check up on it again. Your thoughts are a perfect example. You may feel that your new habit of having uplifting thoughts is well set, and you may feel you can stop keeping an eye on it. But, once in a while, depending on what goes on in your life, you may express self-doubt in your thoughts and then the ball is suddenly rolling the wrong way. It is an ongoing process, so go ahead and set a date, as often as you feel it is necessary to keep an eye on your progress. And remember to readjust as necessary.

Use regular journal entries to re-evaluate your goals and objectives. Evaluate at least once a month where you stand. What do you want? What would make you happy in the coming weeks and months? Did you reach a major milestones and forget to take a moment to celebrate? Those moments are so important. Don't be so busy focusing on the next step that you don't spend time congratulating yourself on your wins.

Make a list of everything you succeeded at, no matter how small. When you make this list at the end of the week or the month, always put more positive than negative items down; it will help you see and feel that you are moving forward. For example, on weekends, when I do my recap of the week, I put in ten or more positive things I did or accomplished and list only three that I need to work on.

Have you almost reached a goal but are not satisfied? Analyze why you feel this way and improve your goal so that when you reach it, you will feel amazing. For example, you may be at your goal weight, but you are still neurotic about your relationship with food and still unhappy. Take some time to analyze the situation and ask yourself all those questions we covered in this book. It is important to know and to understand all the way down to your core that the journey is more important than the end result. But when you do reach your goal allow yourself to feel amazing about it!

Find out which season you are in your life. Are you in winter, fall, spring, or summer? There is a great book from William Bridges called *Transitions: Making Sense of Life's Changes* that can help you find out more about the season you are in. Depending on the season, you will take different actions. When you are in winter, you'll require some down time and it may not be the right time to move. However, action gets the energy going. I wanted to take two months off work to sleep because I was exhausted. My brain was tired from all the noise. But for me, that move would have been wrong; I would have entered depression. I needed to keep moving; I needed to take some form of action however small. I did and eventually, I saw the lights of spring.

Your goal is to keep healthy, be at a healthy weight, and to have a healthy relationship with food. Achieving this from the inside out will take time—it can't be accomplished through a fad diet. Be patient. You may not always see how this kind of work improves you on the inside, but it does. And that is why you have to keep a close eye on things by reviewing your actions and thoughts at the end of each week by writing it down in your journal. Don't be tempted to take the quick road to weight loss. It will land you back at square one again. You'll be thinner, but you'll still be unhappy. Break the cycle once and for all.

Slow down. Stop running everywhere. When you walk slower, move slower, and breathe deeply, it makes you feel calmer. It also helps you to listen, really listen, to your body and your inner self. It may take some effort at first to add more time in your day, but it is worth it. I have now committed myself to take 1 or 2 hrs for me everyday. Some time for physical training and some time for meditating. The benefits are amazing. If you cannot set aside 1 or 2 hours than here are some tricks: if you need to be somewhere and it will take twenty minutes to get there, plan for thirty and take your time, breathe and meditate actively; or brush your teeth slower or empty the dishwasher slower. Make a conscious effort to slow down and you will notice that you are calmer. And if you are calmer, you won't need to reach for the junk food because you are listening to what is going on.

Here is one final exercise that I find useful. Write your own obituary; a detailed one. Write it *as-if* you knew that you were going to die of old age at 105 years old and write everything you want to accomplish for the rest of your life. And when you read it, you view it *as-if* it has already happen and you are tremendously happy and satisfied with your life.

In conclusion, recognize that you are not done. You will never be done. I will never be done, and, believe it or not, that is a great thing. Improving who you are and who you want to be on a daily and weekly basis can be fun. It can also be an amazing source of energy—something to always pull you forward. So don't see losing weight as, "Oh, my God! When will this be done?" because this is how you grow, this is your life and it will be done only when you are dead! See every day as an opportunity to do something for yourself because you are worth it and because you are the most important person in your life. Yes, you are and yes, I am.

Acknowledgments

Peter, thank you for your constant support and belief that I can be the best I can be. You are my rock.

Thanks Cathy for your friendship and support. It means the world to me.

I want to thank my mom for being a great role model of strength and class. Mom, I miss you.

Thank you Stephanie and Judith for the copy editing of my book. You did a great job.

I am so grateful to my amazing supporters and friends who have read the book and suggested great changes to improve it.

Suggested Readings, Web Sites, and Tools

Barnes, Sophie L : www.helpheretoday.com

Bridges, William. *Transitions: Making Sense of Life's Changes*

Cameron, Julia. *The Artist's Way*

Canfield, Jack and Janet Switzer. *The Success Principles: How to Get from Where You Are to Where You Want to Be*

Fitbit pedometer. www.fitbit.com

Myss, Caroline. *Anatomy of the Spirit*

Robbins, Tony. http://www.tonyrobbins.com

Roberge, Michèle. *Tant d'hiver au coeur du changement*

www.ingramcontent.com/pod-product-compliance
Lightning Source LLC
Chambersburg PA
CBHW070651290526
45790CB00001B/277